WHAT OTHERS ARE SAYING ...

"Weinstein approaches nutrition and exercise with military precision."

- The Miami Herald

"Bob spells out simple ways that need no gym or fancy gym equipment to get and stay in good physical shape ...."

- Ursula E. Hanks

"Highly motivating and interesting method for self-help in health & fitness. It concentrates on the affordable method, instead of spending much money on expensive equipment and gym fees to get fit."

- Priscilla Smith

Col. Weinstein has been featured as a health and fitness expert:

Baptist Health Hospitals

Fitness Magazine

The History Channel

Fox Sports Net

The Washington Times

The Las Vegas Tribune

Eurosport, the largest European satellite and cable network

Gold Coast Magazine

Tropical Life Magazine

The Sun-sentinel

The Miami Herald

I0026705

"Most people never run far enough on their first wind to find out they've got a second. Give your dreams all you've got and you'll be amazed at the energy that comes out of you."

- William James, Psychologist and Author

FOOD AND FITNESS JOURNAL

ACHIEVE YOUR GOALS IN NINETY DAYS

By Lt. Col. Bob Weinstein, USAR-Ret.
Boot Camp Fitness Instructor

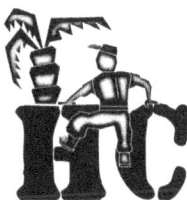

Health Colonel Publishing

"Write it Down and You Will Succeed!"

This journal belongs to

_____

Food and Fitness Journal - Achieve Your Goals in Ninety Days
By Lt. Col. Bob Weinstein, USAR-Ret.
(Lt. Col. Joseph R. Weinstein, USAR-Ret.)
www .TheHealthColonel.com
Categories: health and fitness, weight loss, exercise journals, food diary

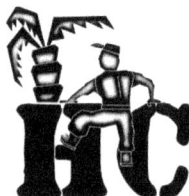

Health Colonel Publishing
The Health Colonel Series™

Weinstein, Bob.
Weinstein, Joseph
Food and Fitness Journal - Achieve Your Goals in Ninety Days: the health colonel's success
journal / by Bob Weinstein (Joseph Weinstein).– 1st ed.
ISBN-13: 978-1-935759-03-4 (trade pbk. : alk. Paper)
1. Fitness, Weight Loss–United States. I. Weinstein, Bob. Weinstein, Joseph. II. Title. III.
Title: Food and Fitness Journal

Printed in the United States

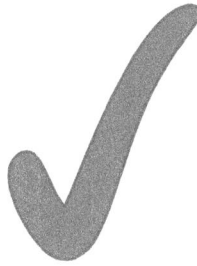

Write
down
what you
eat and drink
and weigh
yourself regularly
and you will have
greater success losing
those extra pounds.

Dedication

This book is dedicated to
my loving wife, Grit
who supports me in all that I do.

Acknowledgements

A big thank you to all the
beach boot camp recruits on Fort Lauderdale Beach.
You remain a constant source of inspiration.
You demonstrate that it is possible to combine
fun, friendship and exercise.
May you enjoy a healthy and happy life.

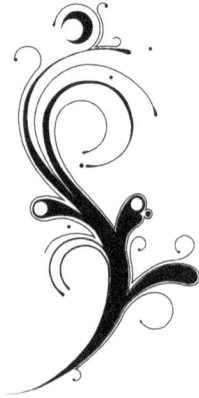

CONTENTS

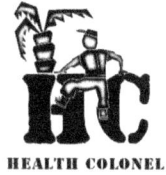

PART ONE - Getting Started

PART TWO - 90 Day Journal with Inspirational Quotes

"Most people spend more time and energy going around problems than in trying to solve them."

- Henry Ford

Ground Rules to Succeed

1. Know the who, what, why, how, when and where.

Get your plan together and don't worry if it is incomplete. Action is preceded by planning. Some of the details of that goal are gathered while you are on the move to achieve your goals. This journal serves the purpose of helping you to keep the who, what, why, how, when and where covered as you pursue your journaling journey to better health. A poem by Rudyard Kipling says it best:

> *"I keep six honest serving-men*
> *(They taught me all I knew.)*
> *Their names are What and Why and When*
> *And How and Where and Who."*

2. Never give up if the cause is worthy.

Better health is a worthy cause. Therefore, never ever give up. Sir Winston Churchill said it best:

> *"Never give in--never, never, never, never, in nothing great or small, large or petty, never give in except to convictions of honour and good sense."*

3. Go around, through, over and/or under all obstacles.

There will be obstacles along the way. Deal with them and overcome them. There will be interruptions, set-backs, and thoughts of "I don't feel like it." that will invade the mind.

4. Inject Vitamin "D" for Discipline into your plan.

Take a good dose of D for discipline to keep you on track when you don't feel like it.

5. Take personal responsibility for your situation.

Never blame external circumstances or other people. That will keep you empowered to improve.

Free Resources
On Exercise And Healthy Eating

Health, Nutrition and Exercise
www.hhs.gov
US Dept of Health and Human Services

Exercise Activity for Everyone
US National Library of Medicine and National Institute of Health
www.nlm.nih.gov/medlineplus

Exercise for Older Adults
US Dept. of Health and Human Services
www.nihseniorhealth.gov

Dietary Guidelines for Americans
US Dept. of Agriculture
www.cnpp.usda.gov
www.mypyramid.gov

Free BMI Calculators
The President's Challenge
President's Council on Physical Fitness and Sports
www.presidentschallenge.org
www.nhlbisupport.com/bmi/
www.fitness.gov

Look up Calories or Nutrients in Food
www.nal.usda.gov/fnic/foodcomp/search

Youth Weight Management
www.nutrition.gov

Menu Planner
National Heart, Lung and Blood Institute
http://hp2010.nhlbihin.net/menuplanner/menu.cgi

Goals - Three-Step Action Plan

➤ **Acknowledge and recognize that there is a problem.**

Have your "deviant" eating habits become a lifestyle? Acknowledging and recognizing the problem appears to be easy to accomplish. It is easy because there is no action required other than acknowledgement and recognition of eating too many bad food choices and too much food. As Albert Einstein once said, *"Insanity is doing the same thing over and over again and expecting a different result."* However, there is more to this. If we are acknowledging and recognizing the problem with the forethought that no action is required, it is bogus and does not count. It is not genuine. Motives do matter and the motive with forethought that no action is required will not bring about the positive change you are looking for.

➤ ➤ **Decide when and how you are going to take action.**

As I jokingly but seriously mention during my fitness training sessions, there are only two things you need to control, your right and your left hand. Because that is how the food and drink you are consuming gets into your body. Start writing down what you are doing in the eating and exercise departments of your life. *Decide when you will start and how you will take action.*

➤ ➤ ➤ **Take action.**

Get up in the morning and start writing down all that you eat and drink. Write down your exercising routines. Add some additional tools for the task, measuring cups and spoons. Instead of two tablespoons of olive oil on your brown rice dish, only use one. Instead of 2 cups of cooked rice, now use the measuring cup and add one cup. Increase the amount of vegetables and measure 2/3 cup of black beans instead of the usual one plus cup. Significantly reduce the calories while increasing the quality. When eating out, the strategy changes. You already know the portions sizes are too big and the menu will tempt you with many choices. You need to decide before you set foot into the restaurant to be portion size conscious and watch the fat and sugar intake. If you order a full meal, you need to have half of it placed in a doggy bag before it gets to your table. You can also share it or order an appetizer.

Body Mass Index (BMI)

The body mass index (BMI) measures the body based on a person's weight and height. BMI is an indicator of the propensity for disease. It doesn't measure the percentage of body fat. BMI is an easy measurement. There are many online calculators so you can quickly find out what your BMI is. Go to Diabetes.com and you will find a free calculator.

BMI calculation formula:
BMI = mass (kg) / (height (m))^2

BMI OR BODY MASS INDEX VALUES

Underweight: Below 18.5
Healthy weight: 18.5 to 24.9
Overweight: 25 to 29.9
Obese: 30 or higher

Go to Diabetes.org, type in "BMI calculator" under "search" and then calculate your BMI.

Mind Set

Pursuing your goals of healthy eating and regular exercise is where your mind needs to be . The truth is losing weight and getting in shape have nothing to do with eating and exercise and have everything to do with how you think. Change your way of thinking and your healthy lifestyle will be the result.

Some important questions to ask to get into the right mind set:

☑ Do you eat foods that enhance your performance and health?

☑ Do you exercise on a daily basis?

☑ Do you specifically work on improving your character and values on a daily basis?

☑ Do you focus on helping others?

☑ Do you encourage or discourage others on a daily basis?

☑ Do you encourage or discourage yourself to lead a healthy lifestyle?

Life is not primarily about fitness, exercise and nutrition. The questions are designed to put you on a values-based program. Such a program helps you to keep your priorities straight.

Basal Metabolic Rate (BMR)

BMR, simply stated, is the caloric expenditure necessary to maintain the function of the vital organs in the body. Your body is essentially at rest and performing no other activities other than keeping the body functioning. Your BMR changes, as a rule, as you age. That means it usually slows. We often talk of a slowed metabolism as we age. Physical activity may increase your BMR and , then again, it may not.

You can get a rough estimate of your BMR by visiting one of the free online BMR calculators. Perform a Google search for "BMR calculator" and you will find one.

My BMR is approximately 1,550 which means that my body needs to burn about 1,550 calories at rest to stay alive. I am 5'8' tall, weigh 165 pounds and am 59 years old.

BMR Formula

Women: BMR = 655 + (4.35 x weight in pounds) + (4.7 x height in inches) - (4.7 x age in years)

Men: BMR = 66 + (6.23 x weight in pounds) + (12.7 x height in inches) - (6.8 x age in year)

Metric
Women: BMR = 655 + (9.6 x weight in kilos) + (1.8 x height in cm) - (4.7 x age in years)

Men: BMR = 66 + (13.7 x weight in kilos) + (5 x height in cm) - (6.8 x age in years)

Take Your Body Measurements

A quick and simple way to measure loss of body fat is to take body measurements with a measuring tape every four weeks as a part of your program. You will need a buddy to take the measurements for you. Always take body measurements on the right side of your body. We will limit the measurements to the following body parts so that you have some fast and easy indicators of your progress. Also, since you will probably be clothed for these measurements, make sure that you are wearing the same clothing for each of the measurements to ensure an accurate measurement of progress. The measurements should be taken at the same time of day, and not just after a meal or a vigorous exercise session.

Measure these body parts:

❖ NECK CIRCUMFERENCE

Your arms are relaxed at your sides in the standing position, and your neck is relaxed. Measure the smallest circumference of your neck, and note the number of inches.

❖ ARM

Measure the arm circumference with the subject standing upright, shoulders relaxed, and the right arm extended out to the side and parallel to the ground. It is important to be certain that the muscle of the arm is not flexed or tightened, which could yield a larger and inaccurate reading. Your buddy will stand facing your right side. Place the tape around the largest part of the bicep/tricep and measure.

❖ CHEST CIRCUMFERENCE

Your arms are relaxed and at your sides. Your buddy takes the measuring tape under your arms and around your chest where the nipples are. Relax your breathing during this measurement.

❖ ABDOMINAL CIRCUMFERENCE

Measure abdominal circumference against the skin at the belly button. Arms are relaxed at the sides. Take a relaxed exhale and have your buddy take the measurement.

❖ WAIST CIRCUMFERENCE

To measure your waist circumference, place a tape measure around your abdominal region just above your hip bone. Be sure that the tape is firm but not too tight. Slowly exhale and take the measurement.

❖ ILIAC CIRCUMFERENCE

Stand and find where your upper pelvic bones protrude the most; you can feel for them on either side of your waist. Measure the circumference at this point. It could be about two inches below the navel (belly button), but can vary from person to person.

❖ HIP CIRCUMFERENCE

Stand and find the area of your body below your navel where you are the widest. This area can vary greatly from person to person. Wrap the tape measure around your body and take the measurement.

❖ CALF CIRCUMFERENCE

You're in the standing position. Relax your right leg and put your weight on your left leg. Now measure the calf circumference of the right at the widest point.

Portion Sizes

GRAIN PRODUCTS

1 Serving Looks Like . . .
1 cup of cereal flakes = fist
1 pancake = compact disc
½ cup of cooked
rice, pasta, or potato = ½ baseball
1 slice of bread = cassette tape
1 piece of cornbread = bar of soap

VEGETABLES AND FRUIT

1 Serving Looks Like . . .
1 cup of salad greens = baseball
1 baked potato = fist
1 med. fruit = baseball
½ cup of fresh fruit = ½ baseball
¼ cup of raisins = large egg

DAIRY AND CHEESE

1 Serving Looks Like . . .
1½ oz. cheese = 4 stacked dice or 2 cheese slices
½ cup of ice cream = ½ baseball

FATS

1 Serving Looks Like . . .
1 tsp. margarine or spreads = 1 dice

MEAT AND ALTERNATIVES

1 Serving Looks Like . . .
3 oz. meat, fish, and poultry = deck of cards
3 oz. grilled/baked fish = checkbook
2 Tbsp. peanut butter = ping pong ball

Calories

Be Calorie Conscious And Read Labels

Bacon 2 slices 80
Brownie 2 inch square 243
Caesar salad 10 oz w/dressing 520
Carrot, fresh one medium 35
Cheesecake ¼ of 19 oz cake 330
Chicken breast 6 oz 280
Coffee w/sugar Cup 2 tsp sugar 32
Egg white Large 17
Egg with yoke Large 78
Milk 8 oz 160
Oatmeal Cup cooked 147
Oatmeal cookie 113 gr. Einstein's 600
Orange 180 gr. 85
Orange Juice 8 oz 112
Pancakes 2 cakes, 200 gr. 450
Pasta 2 cups cooked 600
Potato chips 1 oz 150
Potato, baked 7 oz 200
Swiss Cheese slice 70
Tortilla chips 4 oz 200
Tuna fish 4.5 oz 120
Watermelon Cup diced 46
White bread 1 slice 67
Yogurt, fruit 8 oz 120

1200 Calorie Menu Example

Breakfast (numbers are calories)
Whole Wheat Bread, 1 med. Slice 70 (1 Bread/Starch)
Jelly, regular, 2 tsp. 30 (1/2 Fruit)
Cereal, Shredded Wheat, 1/2 cup 104 (1 Bread/Starch)
Milk, 1%, 1 cup, 102 (1 Milk)
Orange Juice 3/4 cup, 78 (1 1/2 Fruit)
Coffee, Regular, 1 cup, 5 (Free)
Breakfast Total 389 calories

Lunch
Roast Beef Sandwich:
Whole Wheat Bread, 2 med. Slices, 139 (2 Bread/Starch)
Lean Roast Beef, unseasoned 2 oz, 60, (2 Lean Protein)
Lettuce, 1 Leaf, 1
Tomato 3 med slices, 10, (1 Vegetable)
Mayonnaise, low-calorie, 1 tsps, 15 (1/3 Fat)
Apple, 1 med, 80(1 Fruit)
Water, 1 cup, (Free)
Lunch Total, 305 calories

Dinner
Salmon. 2 oz edible, 103 (2 Lean Protein)
Vegetable oil, 11/2 tsps, 60 (1 1/2 Fat)
Baked Potato, 3/4 med, 100 (1 Bread/Starch)
Margarine, 1 tsp, 34 (1 Fat)
Green Beans seasoned, with margarine, 1/2 cup, 52 (1 Vegetable) (1/2 Fat)
Carrots, seasoned, 35 (1 Vegetable)
White Dinner Roll, 1 sm, 70 (1 Bread/Starch)
Iced Tea, unsweetened, 1 cup, 0(Free)
Water, 2 cups, 0 (Free)
Dinner total, 454 calories

Snack
Popcorn, 2 1/2 cups, 69 (1 Bread/Starch)
Margarine, 3/4 tsp, 30 (3/4 Fat)
Total calories 1247

Physical Fitness Test, Military-style

Push-ups
Crunches or sit-ups
One mile run/walk

❖ PUSH-UPS (KNEE OR REGULAR)

The push-up will test the endurance of your chest, shoulders and triceps. Rest is permitted in the up position of the push-up or by raising your rearward anatomy while in the upward push-up position. Only correct push-ups count. You have two minutes to perform as many as you can. You count the completed repetition in the up position.

❖ CRUNCHES OR SIT-UPS

Choose regular crunches or sit-ups for this event. The sit-up measures the endurance of your abdominals and hip-flexor muscles. Perform as many as you can within two minutes. You will notice that time is really of the essence when performing this event. Keep the pace up as fast as you reasonably can. Only correct repetitions count. Resting is permitted only in the "up" position for the sit-up. There is no resting position for crunches; continue performing them until the two minutes are up, or stop prior to the two minutes if too fatigued to continue.

❖ ONE MILE RUN/WALK

The one-mile run/walk is designed to measure your aerobic fitness and leg endurance. If, however, you do not have a measured one-mile distance, pick an approximate distance with clear beginning and ending landmarks, and always use this course for your measurement of progress. Your objective is to complete this event as fast as you reasonably can.

❖ RECORD YOUR SCORES AND ESTABLISH YOUR FOUR-WEEK GOALS

You may need some help with establishing your goals. If you are out of shape and just starting out, you will find that, with consistency, you will make significant progress with all three events.

❖ HOW TO ESTABLISH FITNESS GOALS

Let's say you completed the one-mile run/walk in 11 minutes. I would expect that with your next test, you will complete the mile run within a range of 9 to 10 minutes, shaving off one to two minutes of your time. You will conduct a test every four weeks for at least four months. As your fitness improves the goals will probably not be that different.

Beginner Workout Plan, example

MONDAY	TUESDAY	WEDNESDAY
Cardio Walk/jog 15 min. Brief stretch	**Cardio** Walk/jog 15 min. Brief stretch	**Cardio** Walk/jog 15 min. Brief stretch
Upper Body 2 sets each: Push-ups 5 Upright row 10 Shoulder Pr. 5 Dips 10 Bicep Curls 10	**Upper Body** 2 sets each: Push-ups 5 Upright row 10 Shoulder Pr. 5 Dips 10 Bicep Curls 10	**Upper Body** 2 sets each: Push-ups 5 Upright row 10 Shoulder Pr. 5 Dips 10 Bicep Curls 10
Lower Body 2 sets each: Squats 20 Stand.Lunges 20 Dirty Dogs 10 Stand.Crunch 20	**Lower Body** 2 sets each: Squats 20 Stand.Lunges 20 Dirty Dogs 10 Stand.Crunch 20	**Lower Body** 2 sets each: Squats 20 Stand.Lunges 20 Dirty Dogs 10 Stand.Crunch 20
Abs 2 sets each: Crunches 50 4-ct. Leg. Lev. 5 Flutter kicks 5	**Abs** 2 sets each: Crunches 50 4-ct. Leg. Lev. 5 Flutter kicks 5	**Abs** 2 sets each: Crunches 50 4-ct. Leg. Lev. 5 Flutter kicks 5
Stretch 3 min. Upper body Lower body	**Stretch** 3 min. Upper body Lower body	**Stretch** 3 min. Upper body Lower body

Beginner Workout Plan, example

THURSDAY	FRIDAY	SATURDAY
Cardio	**Cardio**	**Cardio**
Walk/jog 15 min.	Walk/jog 15 min.	Walk/jog 25 min.
Brief stretch	Brief stretch	Brief stretch
Upper Body	**Upper Body**	**Upper Body**
2 sets each:	2 sets each:	2 sets each:
Push-ups 5	Push-ups 5	Push-ups 5
Upright row 10	Upright row 10	Upright row 10
Shoulder Pr. 5	Shoulder Pr. 5	Shoulder Pr. 5
Dips 10	Dips 10	Dips 10
Bicep Curls 10	Bicep Curls 10	Bicep Curls 10
Lower Body	**Lower Body**	**Lower Body**
2 sets each:	2 sets each:	2 sets each:
Squats 20	Squats 20	Squats 20
Stand.Lunges 20	Stand.Lunges 20	Stand.Lunges 20
Dirty Dogs 10	Dirty Dogs 10	Dirty Dogs 10
Stand.Crunch 20	Stand.Crunch 20	Stand.Crunch 20
Abs	**Abs**	**Abs**
2 sets each:	2 sets each:	2 sets each:
Crunches 50	Crunches 50	Crunches 50
4-ct. Leg. Lev. 5	4-ct. Leg. Lev. 5	4-ct. Leg. Lev. 5
Flutter kicks 5	Flutter kicks 5	Flutter kicks 5
Stretch	**Stretch**	**Stretch**
3 min.	3 min.	3 min.
Upper body	Upper body	Upper body
Lower body	Lower body	Lower body

Lifestyle Change Contract
Values Determine Behavior

Complete your contract for change of lifestyle habit and you will increase your chances of success.

1. I want to change the following lifestyle habit:

2. I want to change this habit for the following reasons:

3. If I changed this habit, I feel I would:

4. The results of the change by me:

5. I plan to make this change in the following manner (list specific steps or action plans for creating this change).

6. My plan for evaluating my success will include:

I agree to discuss further my change in my lifestyle habit with
_____ by
_____ (date).

I agree to discuss with _____
his/her success in changing a lifestyle habit by _____
(date).

_____
Signature of partner

"There are no hopeless situations, there are only people who have grown hopeless about them."

- Clare Boothe Luce

_____ _____
Date   Day of the week

Day #

Your expectations decide your success. ☐

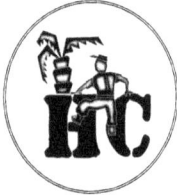

Breakfast	Quantity	Calories	Fat grams	Carb grams	Protein grams	Fiber grams
Breakfast Totals						

Lunch	Quantity	Calories	Fat grams	Carb grams	Protein grams	Fiber grams
Lunch Totals						

Dinner	Quantity	Calories	Fat grams	Carb grams	Protein grams	Fiber grams
Dinner Totals						

M = Morning
A = Afternoon
E = Evening

Weight

Total 8 oz. glasses
of water today:

Snacks	Quantity	Calories	Fat grams	Carbs grams	Protein grams	Fiber grams
Snack Totals						

Vitamins, Meds and other Supplements

		Calories	Fat grams	Carbs grams	Protein grams	Fiber grams
GRAND TOTALS > DAY#						

Physical Fitness

Type	Hours	Reps/Sets	Intensity	Calories Burned

	Bad									Excellent
My Attitude	1	2	3	4	5	6	7	8	9	10
On Track?	1	2	3	4	5	6	7	8	9	10
Belief Meter	1	2	3	4	5	6	7	8	9	10

Day #

Measure it and it will improve.

Breakfast	Quantity	Calories	Fat grams	Carb grams	Protein grams	Fiber grams
Breakfast Totals						

Lunch	Quantity	Calories	Fat grams	Carb grams	Protein grams	Fiber grams
Lunch Totals						

Dinner	Quantity	Calories	Fat grams	Carb grams	Protein grams	Fiber grams
Dinner Totals						

M = Morning
A = Afternoon
E = Evening

Weight

Total 8 oz. glasses
of water today:

Snacks	Quantity	Calories	Fat grams	Carbs grams	Protein grams	Fiber grams
Snack Totals						

Vitamins, Meds and other Supplements

		Calories	Fat grams	Carbs grams	Protein grams	Fiber grams
GRAND TOTALS > DAY#						

Physical Fitness

Type	Hours	Reps/Sets	Intensity	Calories Burned

	Bad									Excellent
My Attitude	1	2	3	4	5	6	7	8	9	10
On Track?	1	2	3	4	5	6	7	8	9	10
Belief Meter	1	2	3	4	5	6	7	8	9	10

_____ _____
Date   Day of the week

_____
Day #

Don't quit! Don't give up!

Breakfast	Quantity	Calories	Fat grams	Carb grams	Protein grams	Fiber grams
Breakfast Totals						

Lunch	Quantity	Calories	Fat grams	Carb grams	Protein grams	Fiber grams
Lunch Totals						

Dinner	Quantity	Calories	Fat grams	Carb grams	Protein grams	Fiber grams
Dinner Totals						

M = Morning
A = Afternoon
E = Evening

Weight

Total 8 oz. glasses
of water today:

Snacks	Quantity	Calories	Fat grams	Carbs grams	Protein grams	Fiber grams
Snack Totals						

Vitamins, Meds and other Supplements

		Calories	Fat grams	Carbs grams	Protein grams	Fiber grams
GRAND TOTALS > **DAY#**						

Physical Fitness

Type	Hours	Reps/Sets	Intensity	Calories Burned

	Bad									Excellent
My Attitude	1	2	3	4	5	6	7	8	9	10
On Track?	1	2	3	4	5	6	7	8	9	10
Belief Meter	1	2	3	4	5	6	7	8	9	10

_____
Day #

If you fall down, get back up.

Breakfast	Quantity	Calories	Fat grams	Carb grams	Protein grams	Fiber grams
Breakfast Totals						

Lunch	Quantity	Calories	Fat grams	Carb grams	Protein grams	Fiber grams
Lunch Totals						

Dinner	Quantity	Calories	Fat grams	Carb grams	Protein grams	Fiber grams
Dinner Totals						

M = Morning
A = Afternoon
E = Evening

Weight

Total 8 oz. glasses
of water today:

Snacks	Quantity	Calories	Fat grams	Carbs grams	Protein grams	Fiber grams
Snack Totals						

Vitamins, Meds and other Supplements

		Calories	Fat grams	Carbs grams	Protein grams	Fiber grams
GRAND TOTALS > **DAY#**						

Physical Fitness

Type	Hours	Reps/Sets	Intensity	Calories Burned

	Bad									Excellent
My Attitude	1	2	3	4	5	6	7	8	9	10
On Track?	1	2	3	4	5	6	7	8	9	10
Belief Meter	1	2	3	4	5	6	7	8	9	10

Date _____   Day of the week _____

___
Day #

Take it one step at a time.

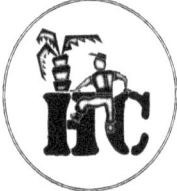

Breakfast	Quantity	Calories	Fat grams	Carb grams	Protein grams	Fiber grams
Breakfast Totals						

Lunch	Quantity	Calories	Fat grams	Carb grams	Protein grams	Fiber grams
Lunch Totals						

Dinner	Quantity	Calories	Fat grams	Carb grams	Protein grams	Fiber grams
Dinner Totals						

M = Morning
A = Afternoon
E = Evening

Weight

Total 8 oz. glasses of water today:

Snacks	Quantity	Calories	Fat grams	Carbs grams	Protein grams	Fiber grams
Snack Totals						

Vitamins, Meds and other Supplements

		Calories	Fat grams	Carbs grams	Protein grams	Fiber grams
GRAND TOTALS > DAY#						

Physical Fitness

Type	Hours	Reps/Sets	Intensity	Calories Burned

My Attitude	800	1	2	3	4	5	6	7	8	9	Excellent 10
On Track?		1	2	3	4	5	6	7	8	9	10
Belief Meter		1	2	3	4	5	6	7	8	9	10

_____
Day #

Decide and then take action.

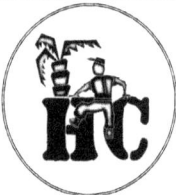

Breakfast	Quantity	Calories	Fat grams	Carb grams	Protein grams	Fiber grams
Breakfast Totals						

Lunch	Quantity	Calories	Fat grams	Carb grams	Protein grams	Fiber grams
Lunch Totals						

Dinner	Quantity	Calories	Fat grams	Carb grams	Protein grams	Fiber grams
Dinner Totals						

M = Morning
A = Afternoon
E = Evening

Weight

Total 8 oz. glasses
of water today:

Snacks	Quantity	Calories	Fat grams	Carbs grams	Protein grams	Fiber grams
Snack Totals						

Vitamins, Meds and other Supplements

		Calories	Fat grams	Carbs grams	Protein grams	Fiber grams
GRAND TOTALS > DAY#						

Physical Fitness

Type	Hours	Reps/Sets	Intensity	Calories Burned

	Bad									Excellent
My Attitude	1	2	3	4	5	6	7	8	9	10
On Track?	1	2	3	4	5	6	7	8	9	10
Belief Meter	1	2	3	4	5	6	7	8	9	10

Day #

Plan like you've already succeeded.

Breakfast	Quantity	Calories	Fat grams	Carb grams	Protein grams	Fiber grams
Breakfast Totals						

Lunch	Quantity	Calories	Fat grams	Carb grams	Protein grams	Fiber grams
Lunch Totals						

Dinner	Quantity	Calories	Fat grams	Carb grams	Protein grams	Fiber grams
Dinner Totals						

Weight

Total 8 oz. glasses
of water today:

Snacks	Quantity	Calories	Fat grams	Carbs grams	Protein grams	Fiber grams
Snack Totals						

Vitamins, Meds and other Supplements

		Calories	Fat grams	Carbs grams	Protein grams	Fiber grams
GRAND TOTALS > **DAY#**						

Physical Fitness

Type	Hours	Reps/Sets	Intensity	Calories Burned

	Bad									Excellent
My Attitude	1	2	3	4	5	6	7	8	9	10
On Track?	1	2	3	4	5	6	7	8	9	10
Belief Meter	1	2	3	4	5	6	7	8	9	10

___
Day #

Make peace with your past.

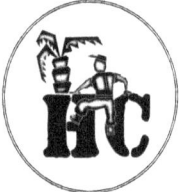

Breakfast	Quantity	Calories	Fat grams	Carb grams	Protein grams	Fiber grams
Breakfast Totals						

Lunch	Quantity	Calories	Fat grams	Carb grams	Protein grams	Fiber grams
Lunch Totals						

Dinner	Quantity	Calories	Fat grams	Carb grams	Protein grams	Fiber grams
Dinner Totals						

Weight

Total 8 oz. glasses of water today:

Snacks	Quantity	Calories	Fat grams	Carbs grams	Protein grams	Fiber grams
Snack Totals						

Vitamins, Meds and other Supplements

		Calories	Fat grams	Carbs grams	Protein grams	Fiber grams
GRAND TOTALS > DAY#						

Physical Fitness

Type	Hours	Reps/Sets	Intensity	Calories Burned

	Dull									Excellent
My Attitude	1	2	3	4	5	6	7	8	9	10
On Track?	1	2	3	4	5	6	7	8	9	10
Belief Meter	1	2	3	4	5	6	7	8	9	10

_____ _____
Date   Day of the week

Day #

You will succeed as much as you believe.

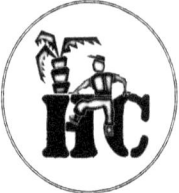

Breakfast	Quantity	Calories	Fat grams	Carb grams	Protein grams	Fiber grams
Breakfast Totals						

Lunch	Quantity	Calories	Fat grams	Carb grams	Protein grams	Fiber grams
Lunch Totals						

Dinner	Quantity	Calories	Fat grams	Carb grams	Protein grams	Fiber grams
Dinner Totals						

M = Morning
A = Afternoon
E = Evening

Weight

Total 8 oz. glasses of water today:

Snacks	Quantity	Calories	Fat grams	Carbs grams	Protein grams	Fiber grams
Snack Totals						

Vitamins, Meds and other Supplements

		Calories	Fat grams	Carbs grams	Protein grams	Fiber grams
GRAND TOTALS > DAY#						

Physical Fitness

Type	Hours	Reps/Sets	Intensity	Calories Burned

	Bad									Excellent
My Attitude	1	2	3	4	5	6	7	8	9	10
On Track?	1	2	3	4	5	6	7	8	9	10
Belief Meter	1	2	3	4	5	6	7	8	9	10

Date _____   Day of the week _____

Day # ____

How far you go is how far you think.

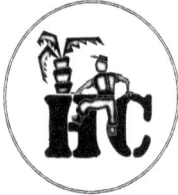

Breakfast	Quantity	Calories	Fat grams	Carb grams	Protein grams	Fiber grams
Breakfast Totals						

Lunch	Quantity	Calories	Fat grams	Carb grams	Protein grams	Fiber grams
Lunch Totals						

Dinner	Quantity	Calories	Fat grams	Carb grams	Protein grams	Fiber grams
Dinner Totals						

M = Morning
A = Afternoon
E = Evening

Weight

Total 8 oz. glasses
of water today:

Snacks	Quantity	Calories	Fat grams	Carbs grams	Protein grams	Fiber grams
Snack Totals						

Vitamins, Meds and other Supplements

		Calories	Fat grams	Carbs grams	Protein grams	Fiber grams
GRAND TOTALS > **DAY#**						

Physical Fitness

Type	Hours	Reps/Sets	Intensity	Calories Burned

	Bad									Excellent
My Attitude	1	2	3	4	5	6	7	8	9	10
On Track?	1	2	3	4	5	6	7	8	9	10
Belief Meter	1	2	3	4	5	6	7	8	9	10

_____ _____
Date   Day of the week

Day #

Get up and show up!

Breakfast	Quantity	Calories	Fat grams	Carb grams	Protein grams	Fiber grams
Breakfast Totals						

Lunch	Quantity	Calories	Fat grams	Carb grams	Protein grams	Fiber grams
Lunch Totals						

Dinner	Quantity	Calories	Fat grams	Carb grams	Protein grams	Fiber grams
Dinner Totals						

Weight

Total 8 oz. glasses
of water today:

Snacks	Quantity	Calories	Fat grams	Carbs grams	Protein grams	Fiber grams
Snack Totals						

Vitamins, Meds and other Supplements

		Calories	Fat grams	Carbs grams	Protein grams	Fiber grams
GRAND TOTALS > **DAY#**						

Physical Fitness

Type	Hours	Reps/Sets	Intensity	Calories Burned

	Bad									Excellent
My Attitude	1	2	3	4	5	6	7	8	9	10
On Track?	1	2	3	4	5	6	7	8	9	10
Belief Meter	1	2	3	4	5	6	7	8	9	10

	Date				Day of the week	

Day #

Motive always matters.

Breakfast	Quantity	Calories	Fat grams	Carb grams	Protein grams	Fiber grams
Breakfast Totals						
Lunch	Quantity	Calories	Fat grams	Carb grams	Protein grams	Fiber grams
Lunch Totals						
Dinner	Quantity	Calories	Fat grams	Carb grams	Protein grams	Fiber grams
Dinner Totals						

Weight

Total 8 oz. glasses of water today:

Snacks	Quantity	Calories	Fat grams	Carbs grams	Protein grams	Fiber grams
Snack Totals						

Vitamins, Meds and other Supplements

		Calories	Fat grams	Carbs grams	Protein grams	Fiber grams
GRAND TOTALS > DAY#						

Physical Fitness

Type	Hours	Reps/Sets	Intensity	Calories Burned

	Bad									Excellent
My Attitude	1	2	3	4	5	6	7	8	9	10
On Track?	1	2	3	4	5	6	7	8	9	10
Belief Meter	1	2	3	4	5	6	7	8	9	10

_____ _____
Date   Day of the week

_____
Day #

Get amnesia about what you cannot do.

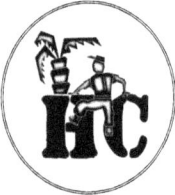

Breakfast	Quantity	Calories	Fat grams	Carb grams	Protein grams	Fiber grams
Breakfast Totals						

Lunch	Quantity	Calories	Fat grams	Carb grams	Protein grams	Fiber grams
Lunch Totals						

Dinner	Quantity	Calories	Fat grams	Carb grams	Protein grams	Fiber grams
Dinner Totals						

M = Morning
A = Afternoon
E = Evening

Weight

Total 8 oz. glasses
of water today:

Snacks	Quantity	Calories	Fat grams	Carbs grams	Protein grams	Fiber grams
Snack Totals						

Vitamins, Meds and other Supplements

		Calories	Fat grams	Carbs grams	Protein grams	Fiber grams
GRAND TOTALS > DAY#						

Physical Fitness

Type	Hours	Reps/Sets	Intensity	Calories Burned

	Bad									Excellent
My Attitude	1	2	3	4	5	6	7	8	9	10
On Track?	1	2	3	4	5	6	7	8	9	10
Belief Meter	1	2	3	4	5	6	7	8	9	10

_____ Date   _____ Day of the week

Day #

Do what is right, not what is comfortable.

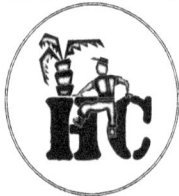

Breakfast	Quantity	Calories	Fat grams	Carb grams	Protein grams	Fiber grams
Breakfast Totals						
Lunch	Quantity	Calories	Fat grams	Carb grams	Protein grams	Fiber grams
Lunch Totals						
Dinner	Quantity	Calories	Fat grams	Carb grams	Protein grams	Fiber grams
Dinner Totals						

Weight

Total 8 oz. glasses
of water today:

Snacks	Quantity	Calories	Fat grams	Carbs grams	Protein grams	Fiber grams
Snack Totals						

Vitamins, Meds and other Supplements

		Calories	Fat grams	Carbs grams	Protein grams	Fiber grams
GRAND TOTALS > **DAY#**						

Physical Fitness

Type	Hours	Reps/Sets	Intensity	Calories Burned

	Bad									Excellent
My Attitude	1	2	3	4	5	6	7	8	9	10
On Track?	1	2	3	4	5	6	7	8	9	10
Belief Meter	1	2	3	4	5	6	7	8	9	10

_____ _____
Date   Day of the week

_____
Day #

**If the cause is worthy,
never give up.**

Breakfast	Quantity	Calories	Fat grams	Carb grams	Protein grams	Fiber grams
Breakfast Totals						

Lunch	Quantity	Calories	Fat grams	Carb grams	Protein grams	Fiber grams
Lunch Totals						

Dinner	Quantity	Calories	Fat grams	Carb grams	Protein grams	Fiber grams
Dinner Totals						

Weight

Total 8 oz. glasses of water today:

Snacks	Quantity	Calories	Fat grams	Carbs grams	Protein grams	Fiber grams
Snack Totals						

Vitamins, Meds and other Supplements

		Calories	Fat grams	Carbs grams	Protein grams	Fiber grams
GRAND TOTALS > DAY#						

Physical Fitness

Type	Hours	Reps/Sets	Intensity	Calories Burned

	Bad									Excellent
My Attitude	1	2	3	4	5	6	7	8	9	10
On Track?	1	2	3	4	5	6	7	8	9	10
Belief Meter	1	2	3	4	5	6	7	8	9	10

_____ _____
Date   Day of the week

_____
Day #

Do what you say you're going to do.

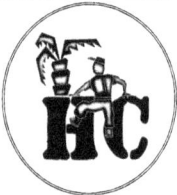

Breakfast	Quantity	Calories	Fat grams	Carb grams	Protein grams	Fiber grams
Breakfast Totals						
Lunch	Quantity	Calories	Fat grams	Carb grams	Protein grams	Fiber grams
Lunch Totals						
Dinner	Quantity	Calories	Fat grams	Carb grams	Protein grams	Fiber grams
Dinner Totals						

M = Morning
A = Afternoon
E = Evening

Weight

Total 8 oz. glasses
of water today:

Snacks	Quantity	Calories	Fat grams	Carbs grams	Protein grams	Fiber grams
Snack Totals						

Vitamins, Meds and other Supplements

		Calories	Fat grams	Carbs grams	Protein grams	Fiber grams
GRAND TOTALS > DAY#						

Physical Fitness

Type	Hours	Reps/Sets	Intensity	Calories Burned

	Bad									Excellent
My Attitude	1	2	3	4	5	6	7	8	9	10
On Track?	1	2	3	4	5	6	7	8	9	10
Belief Meter	1	2	3	4	5	6	7	8	9	10

_____   _____
Date   Day of the week

_____
Day #

Overeating 400 calories a day equals 146,000 calories per year.

Breakfast	Quantity	Calories	Fat grams	Carb grams	Protein grams	Fiber grams
Breakfast Totals						
Lunch	Quantity	Calories	Fat grams	Carb grams	Protein grams	Fiber grams
Lunch Totals						
Dinner	Quantity	Calories	Fat grams	Carb grams	Protein grams	Fiber grams
Dinner Totals						

M = Morning
A = Afternoon
E = Evening

Weight

Total 8 oz. glasses
of water today:

Snacks	Quantity	Calories	Fat grams	Carbs grams	Protein grams	Fiber grams
Snack Totals						

Vitamins, Meds and other Supplements

		Calories	Fat grams	Carbs grams	Protein grams	Fiber grams
GRAND TOTALS > DAY#						

Physical Fitness

Type	Hours	Reps/Sets	Intensity	Calories Burned

	Bad									Excellent
My Attitude	1	2	3	4	5	6	7	8	9	10
On Track?	1	2	3	4	5	6	7	8	9	10
Belief Meter	1	2	3	4	5	6	7	8	9	10

_____   _____
Date   Day of the week

_____
Day #

Overeating 400 calories a day equates to 40 pounds of fat in one year.

Breakfast	Quantity	Calories	Fat grams	Carb grams	Protein grams	Fiber grams
Breakfast Totals						

Lunch	Quantity	Calories	Fat grams	Carb grams	Protein grams	Fiber grams
Lunch Totals						

Dinner	Quantity	Calories	Fat grams	Carb grams	Protein grams	Fiber grams
Dinner Totals						

M = Morning
A = Afternoon
E = Evening

Weight

Total 8 oz. glasses
of water today:

Snacks	Quantity	Calories	Fat grams	Carbs grams	Protein grams	Fiber grams
Snack Totals						

Vitamins, Meds and other Supplements

		Calories	Fat grams	Carbs grams	Protein grams	Fiber grams
GRAND TOTALS > DAY#						

Physical Fitness

Type	Hours	Reps/Sets	Intensity	Calories Burned

	Bad									Excellent
My Attitude	1	2	3	4	5	6	7	8	9	10
On Track?	1	2	3	4	5	6	7	8	9	10
Belief Meter	1	2	3	4	5	6	7	8	9	10

_____ _____
Date   Day of the week

Day #

Adversity is the ultimate test of character.

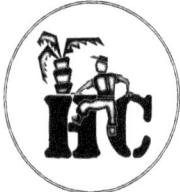

Breakfast	Quantity	Calories	Fat grams	Carb grams	Protein grams	Fiber grams
Breakfast Totals						

Lunch	Quantity	Calories	Fat grams	Carb grams	Protein grams	Fiber grams
Lunch Totals						

Dinner	Quantity	Calories	Fat grams	Carb grams	Protein grams	Fiber grams
Dinner Totals						

Weight

Total 8 oz. glasses
of water today:

Snacks	Quantity	Calories	Fat grams	Carbs grams	Protein grams	Fiber grams
Snack Totals						

Vitamins, Meds and other Supplements

		Calories	Fat grams	Carbs grams	Protein grams	Fiber grams
GRAND TOTALS > **DAY#**						

Physical Fitness

Type	Hours	Reps/Sets	Intensity	Calories Burned

	Bad									Excellent
My Attitude	1	2	3	4	5	6	7	8	9	10
On Track?	1	2	3	4	5	6	7	8	9	10
Belief Meter	1	2	3	4	5	6	7	8	9	10

_____ Date   _____ Day of the week

_____
Day #

Develop a bounce back attitude.

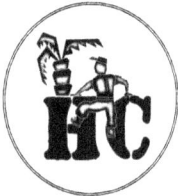

Breakfast	Quantity	Calories	Fat grams	Carb grams	Protein grams	Fiber grams
Breakfast Totals						

Lunch	Quantity	Calories	Fat grams	Carb grams	Protein grams	Fiber grams
Lunch Totals						

Dinner	Quantity	Calories	Fat grams	Carb grams	Protein grams	Fiber grams
Dinner Totals						

M = Morning
A = Afternoon
E = Evening

Weight

Total 8 oz. glasses
of water today:

Snacks	Quantity	Calories	Fat grams	Carbs grams	Protein grams	Fiber grams
Snack Totals						

Vitamins, Meds and other Supplements

		Calories	Fat grams	Carbs grams	Protein grams	Fiber grams
GRAND TOTALS > DAY#						

Physical Fitness

Type	Hours	Reps/Sets	Intensity	Calories Burned

	Bad									Excellent
My Attitude	1	2	3	4	5	6	7	8	9	10
On Track?	1	2	3	4	5	6	7	8	9	10
Belief Meter	1	2	3	4	5	6	7	8	9	10

_____ _____
Date   Day of the week

Day #

Take charge and take responsibility for your life.

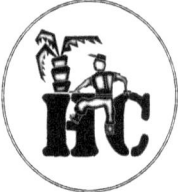

Breakfast	Quantity	Calories	Fat grams	Carb grams	Protein grams	Fiber grams
Breakfast Totals						
Lunch	Quantity	Calories	Fat grams	Carb grams	Protein grams	Fiber grams
Lunch Totals						
Dinner	Quantity	Calories	Fat grams	Carb grams	Protein grams	Fiber grams
Dinner Totals						

M = Morning
A = Afternoon
E = Evening

Weight

Total 8 oz. glasses of water today:

Snacks	Quantity	Calories	Fat grams	Carbs grams	Protein grams	Fiber grams
Snack Totals						

Vitamins, Meds and other Supplements

		Calories	Fat grams	Carbs grams	Protein grams	Fiber grams
GRAND TOTALS > DAY#						

Physical Fitness

Type	Hours	Reps/Sets	Intensity	Calories Burned

	Bad									Excellent
My Attitude	1	2	3	4	5	6	7	8	9	10
On Track?	1	2	3	4	5	6	7	8	9	10
Belief Meter	1	2	3	4	5	6	7	8	9	10

_____ _____
Date   Day of the week

_____
Day #

Discouraging self-talk
will drain you of
positive emotions. ☐

Breakfast	Quantity	Calories	Fat grams	Carb grams	Protein grams	Fiber grams
Breakfast Totals						

Lunch	Quantity	Calories	Fat grams	Carb grams	Protein grams	Fiber grams
Lunch Totals						

Dinner	Quantity	Calories	Fat grams	Carb grams	Protein grams	Fiber grams
Dinner Totals						

M = Morning
A = Afternoon
E = Evening

Weight

Total 8 oz. glasses
of water today:

Snacks	Quantity	Calories	Fat grams	Carbs grams	Protein grams	Fiber grams
Snack Totals						

Vitamins, Meds and other Supplements

		Calories	Fat grams	Carbs grams	Protein grams	Fiber grams
GRAND TOTALS > DAY#						

Physical Fitness

Type	Hours	Reps/Sets	Intensity	Calories Burned

	Bad									Excellent
My Attitude	1	2	3	4	5	6	7	8	9	10
On Track?	1	2	3	4	5	6	7	8	9	10
Belief Meter	1	2	3	4	5	6	7	8	9	10

_____
Day #

Be the one whom others can depend upon. ☐

Breakfast	Quantity	Calories	Fat grams	Carb grams	Protein grams	Fiber grams
Breakfast Totals						

Lunch	Quantity	Calories	Fat grams	Carb grams	Protein grams	Fiber grams
Lunch Totals						

Dinner	Quantity	Calories	Fat grams	Carb grams	Protein grams	Fiber grams
Dinner Totals						

M = Morning
A = Afternoon
E = Evening

Weight

Total 8 oz. glasses of water today:

Snacks	Quantity	Calories	Fat grams	Carbs grams	Protein grams	Fiber grams
Snack Totals						

Vitamins, Meds and other Supplements

		Calories	Fat grams	Carbs grams	Protein grams	Fiber grams
GRAND TOTALS > **DAY#**						

Physical Fitness

Type	Hours	Reps/Sets	Intensity	Calories Burned

	Bad									Excellent
My Attitude	1	2	3	4	5	6	7	8	9	10
On Track?	1	2	3	4	5	6	7	8	9	10
Belief Meter	1	2	3	4	5	6	7	8	9	10

_____   _____
Date   Day of the week

_____
Day #

Seek wisdom in every decision you make.

Breakfast	Quantity	Calories	Fat grams	Carb grams	Protein grams	Fiber grams
Breakfast Totals						
Lunch	Quantity	Calories	Fat grams	Carb grams	Protein grams	Fiber grams
Lunch Totals						
Dinner	Quantity	Calories	Fat grams	Carb grams	Protein grams	Fiber grams
Dinner Totals						

Weight

Total 8 oz. glasses
of water today:

Snacks	Quantity	Calories	Fat grams	Carbs grams	Protein grams	Fiber grams
Snack Totals						

Vitamins, Meds and other Supplements

		Calories	Fat grams	Carbs grams	Protein grams	Fiber grams
GRAND TOTALS > DAY#						

Physical Fitness

Type	Hours	Reps/Sets	Intensity	Calories Burned

	Bad									Excellent
My Attitude	1	2	3	4	5	6	7	8	9	10
On Track?	1	2	3	4	5	6	7	8	9	10
Belief Meter	1	2	3	4	5	6	7	8	9	10

Day #

Find the right questions and you will find the right answers.

Breakfast	Quantity	Calories	Fat grams	Carb grams	Protein grams	Fiber grams
Breakfast Totals						

Lunch	Quantity	Calories	Fat grams	Carb grams	Protein grams	Fiber grams
Lunch Totals						

Dinner	Quantity	Calories	Fat grams	Carb grams	Protein grams	Fiber grams
Dinner Totals						

M = Morning
A = Afternoon
E = Evening

Weight ⬭

Total 8 oz. glasses
of water today:

Snacks	Quantity	Calories	Fat grams	Carbs grams	Protein grams	Fiber grams
Snack Totals						

Vitamins, Meds and other Supplements

		Calories	Fat grams	Carbs grams	Protein grams	Fiber grams
GRAND TOTALS > **DAY#**						

Physical Fitness

Type	Hours	Reps/Sets	Intensity	Calories Burned

	Bad									Excellent
My Attitude	1	2	3	4	5	6	7	8	9	10
On Track?	1	2	3	4	5	6	7	8	9	10
Belief Meter	1	2	3	4	5	6	7	8	9	10

			Date			Day of the week

Day #

Be gracious to everyone no matter how you are treated.

Breakfast	Quantity	Calories	Fat grams	Carb grams	Protein grams	Fiber grams
Breakfast Totals						
Lunch	Quantity	Calories	Fat grams	Carb grams	Protein grams	Fiber grams
Lunch Totals						
Dinner	Quantity	Calories	Fat grams	Carb grams	Protein grams	Fiber grams
Dinner Totals						

M = Morning
A = Afternoon
E = Evening

Weight

Total 8 oz. glasses
of water today:

Snacks	Quantity	Calories	Fat grams	Carbs grams	Protein grams	Fiber grams
Snack Totals						

Vitamins, Meds and other Supplements

		Calories	Fat grams	Carbs grams	Protein grams	Fiber grams
GRAND TOTALS > DAY#						

Physical Fitness

Type	Hours	Reps/Sets	Intensity	Calories Burned

	Bad									Excellent
My Attitude	1	2	3	4	5	6	7	8	9	10
On Track?	1	2	3	4	5	6	7	8	9	10
Belief Meter	1	2	3	4	5	6	7	8	9	10

Day #

The best health insurance is a healthy lifestyle.

Breakfast	Quantity	Calories	Fat grams	Carb grams	Protein grams	Fiber grams
Breakfast Totals						

Lunch	Quantity	Calories	Fat grams	Carb grams	Protein grams	Fiber grams
Lunch Totals						

Dinner	Quantity	Calories	Fat grams	Carb grams	Protein grams	Fiber grams
Dinner Totals						

M = Morning
A = Afternoon
E = Evening

Weight

Total 8 oz. glasses of water today:

Snacks	Quantity	Calories	Fat grams	Carbs grams	Protein grams	Fiber grams
Snack Totals						

Vitamins, Meds and other Supplements

		Calories	Fat grams	Carbs grams	Protein grams	Fiber grams
GRAND TOTALS > DAY#						

Physical Fitness

Type	Hours	Reps/Sets	Intensity	Calories Burned

	Bad									Excellent
My Attitude	1	2	3	4	5	6	7	8	9	10
On Track?	1	2	3	4	5	6	7	8	9	10
Belief Meter	1	2	3	4	5	6	7	8	9	10

_____   _____
Date   Day of the week

_____
Day #

Weight loss is about controlling two things, your left and your right hand.

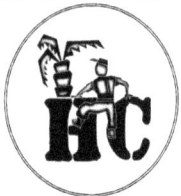

HC

Breakfast	Quantity	Calories	Fat grams	Carb grams	Protein grams	Fiber grams
Breakfast Totals						
Lunch	Quantity	Calories	Fat grams	Carb grams	Protein grams	Fiber grams
Lunch Totals						
Dinner	Quantity	Calories	Fat grams	Carb grams	Protein grams	Fiber grams
Dinner Totals						

Weight

Total 8 oz. glasses
of water today:

Snacks	Quantity	Calories	Fat grams	Carbs grams	Protein grams	Fiber grams
Snack Totals						

Vitamins, Meds and other Supplements

		Calories	Fat grams	Carbs grams	Protein grams	Fiber grams
GRAND TOTALS > **DAY#**						

Physical Fitness

Type	Hours	Reps/Sets	Intensity	Calories Burned

	Bad									Excellent
My Attitude	1	2	3	4	5	6	7	8	9	10
On Track?	1	2	3	4	5	6	7	8	9	10
Belief Meter	1	2	3	4	5	6	7	8	9	10

Day #

Without a struggle there can be no progress.

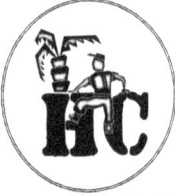

Breakfast	Quantity	Calories	Fat grams	Carb grams	Protein grams	Fiber grams
Breakfast Totals						

Lunch	Quantity	Calories	Fat grams	Carb grams	Protein grams	Fiber grams
Lunch Totals						

Dinner	Quantity	Calories	Fat grams	Carb grams	Protein grams	Fiber grams
Dinner Totals						

Weight

Total 8 oz. glasses of water today:

Snacks	Quantity	Calories	Fat grams	Carbs grams	Protein grams	Fiber grams
Snack Totals						

Vitamins, Meds and other Supplements

		Calories	Fat grams	Carbs grams	Protein grams	Fiber grams
GRAND TOTALS > **DAY#**						

Physical Fitness

Type	Hours	Reps/Sets	Intensity	Calories Burned

	Bad									Excellent
My Attitude	1	2	3	4	5	6	7	8	9	10
On Track?	1	2	3	4	5	6	7	8	9	10
Belief Meter	1	2	3	4	5	6	7	8	9	10

_____   _____
Date   Day of the week

⬭ _____ Day #

Carbs have 4 cal./gram.
Protein has 4 cal./gram.
Alcohol has 7 cal./gram.
Fat has 9 cal./gram.

Breakfast	Quantity	Calories	Fat grams	Carb grams	Protein grams	Fiber grams
Breakfast Totals						

Lunch	Quantity	Calories	Fat grams	Carb grams	Protein grams	Fiber grams
Lunch Totals						

Dinner	Quantity	Calories	Fat grams	Carb grams	Protein grams	Fiber grams
Dinner Totals						

M = Morning
A = Afternoon
E = Evening

Weight

Total 8 oz. glasses
of water today:

Snacks	Quantity	Calories	Fat grams	Carbs grams	Protein grams	Fiber grams
Snack Totals						

Vitamins, Meds and other Supplements

		Calories	Fat grams	Carbs grams	Protein grams	Fiber grams
GRAND TOTALS > **DAY#**						

Physical Fitness

Type	Hours	Reps/Sets	Intensity	Calories Burned

	Bad									Excellent
My Attitude	1	2	3	4	5	6	7	8	9	10
On Track?	1	2	3	4	5	6	7	8	9	10
Belief Meter	1	2	3	4	5	6	7	8	9	10

		Date					Day of the week

Day #

You are the lucky winner of 500 push-ups today.

Breakfast	Quantity	Calories	Fat grams	Carb grams	Protein grams	Fiber grams
Breakfast Totals						

Lunch	Quantity	Calories	Fat grams	Carb grams	Protein grams	Fiber grams
Lunch Totals						

Dinner	Quantity	Calories	Fat grams	Carb grams	Protein grams	Fiber grams
Dinner Totals						

M = Morning
A = Afternoon
E = Evening

Weight

Total 8 oz. glasses
of water today:

Snacks	Quantity	Calories	Fat grams	Carbs grams	Protein grams	Fiber grams
Snack Totals						

Vitamins, Meds and other Supplements

	Calories	Fat grams	Carbs grams	Protein grams	Fiber grams
GRAND TOTALS > DAY#					

Physical Fitness

Type	Hours	Reps/Sets	Intensity	Calories Burned

	Bad									Excellent
My Attitude	1	2	3	4	5	6	7	8	9	10
On Track?	1	2	3	4	5	6	7	8	9	10
Belief Meter	1	2	3	4	5	6	7	8	9	10

____
Day #

If you can't jog, walk.
If you can't walk, crawl.
If you can't crawl, wiggle.

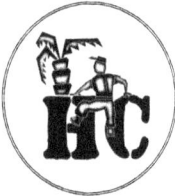

Breakfast	Quantity	Calories	Fat grams	Carb grams	Protein grams	Fiber grams
Breakfast Totals						
Lunch	Quantity	Calories	Fat grams	Carb grams	Protein grams	Fiber grams
Lunch Totals						
Dinner	Quantity	Calories	Fat grams	Carb grams	Protein grams	Fiber grams
Dinner Totals						

M = Morning
A = Afternoon
E = Evening

Weight

Total 8 oz. glasses of water today:

Snacks	Quantity	Calories	Fat grams	Carbs grams	Protein grams	Fiber grams
Snack Totals						

Vitamins, Meds and other Supplements

		Calories	Fat grams	Carbs grams	Protein grams	Fiber grams

GRAND TOTALS > DAY#						

Physical Fitness

Type	Hours	Reps/Sets	Intensity	Calories Burned

	Dud									Excellent
My Attitude	1	2	3	4	5	6	7	8	9	10
On Track?	1	2	3	4	5	6	7	8	9	10
Belief Meter	1	2	3	4	5	6	7	8	9	10

_____ Date   _____ Day of the week

Day #

Do you have peace in your heart?

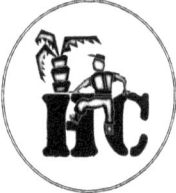

Breakfast	Quantity	Calories	Fat grams	Carb grams	Protein grams	Fiber grams
Breakfast Totals						
Lunch	Quantity	Calories	Fat grams	Carb grams	Protein grams	Fiber grams
Lunch Totals						
Dinner	Quantity	Calories	Fat grams	Carb grams	Protein grams	Fiber grams
Dinner Totals						

M = Morning
A = Afternoon
E = Evening

Weight

Total 8 oz. glasses
of water today:

Snacks	Quantity	Calories	Fat grams	Carbs grams	Protein grams	Fiber grams
Snack Totals						

Vitamins, Meds and other Supplements

		Calories	Fat grams	Carbs grams	Protein grams	Fiber grams
GRAND TOTALS > DAY#						

Physical Fitness

Type	Hours	Reps/Sets	Intensity	Calories Burned

	Bad									Excellent
My Attitude	1	2	3	4	5	6	7	8	9	10
On Track?	1	2	3	4	5	6	7	8	9	10
Belief Meter	1	2	3	4	5	6	7	8	9	10

Day #

Be thankful for everyone and everything you have.

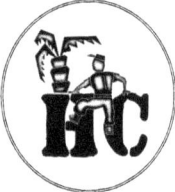

Breakfast	Quantity	Calories	Fat grams	Carb grams	Protein grams	Fiber grams
Breakfast Totals						

Lunch	Quantity	Calories	Fat grams	Carb grams	Protein grams	Fiber grams
Lunch Totals						

Dinner	Quantity	Calories	Fat grams	Carb grams	Protein grams	Fiber grams
Dinner Totals						

Weight

Total 8 oz. glasses of water today:

Snacks	Quantity	Calories	Fat grams	Carbs grams	Protein grams	Fiber grams
Snack Totals						

Vitamins, Meds and other Supplements

		Calories	Fat grams	Carbs grams	Protein grams	Fiber grams
GRAND TOTALS > DAY#						

Physical Fitness

Type	Hours	Reps/Sets	Intensity	Calories Burned

	Bad									Excellent
My Attitude	1	2	3	4	5	6	7	8	9	10
On Track?	1	2	3	4	5	6	7	8	9	10
Belief Meter	1	2	3	4	5	6	7	8	9	10

_____ _____
Date   Day of the week

_____
Day #

Exercise four to six hours per week.

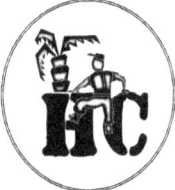

Breakfast	Quantity	Calories	Fat grams	Carb grams	Protein grams	Fiber grams
Breakfast Totals						
Lunch	Quantity	Calories	Fat grams	Carb grams	Protein grams	Fiber grams
Lunch Totals						
Dinner	Quantity	Calories	Fat grams	Carb grams	Protein grams	Fiber grams
Dinner Totals						

M = Morning
A = Afternoon
E = Evening

Weight

Total 8 oz. glasses
of water today:

Snacks	Quantity	Calories	Fat grams	Carbs grams	Protein grams	Fiber grams
Snack Totals						

Vitamins, Meds and other Supplements

		Calories	Fat grams	Carbs grams	Protein grams	Fiber grams
GRAND TOTALS > **DAY#**						

Physical Fitness

Type	Hours	Reps/Sets	Intensity	Calories Burned

	Bad									Excellent
My Attitude	1	2	3	4	5	6	7	8	9	10
On Track?	1	2	3	4	5	6	7	8	9	10
Belief Meter	1	2	3	4	5	6	7	8	9	10

_____ Date   _____ Day of the week

_____ Day #

Cardio is more important than strength or flexibility training.

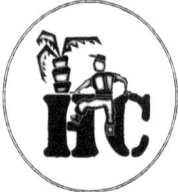

Breakfast	Quantity	Calories	Fat grams	Carb grams	Protein grams	Fiber grams
Breakfast Totals						
Lunch	Quantity	Calories	Fat grams	Carb grams	Protein grams	Fiber grams
Lunch Totals						
Dinner	Quantity	Calories	Fat grams	Carb grams	Protein grams	Fiber grams
Dinner Totals						

Weight

Total 8 oz. glasses
of water today:

Snacks	Quantity	Calories	Fat grams	Carbs grams	Protein grams	Fiber grams
Snack Totals						

Vitamins, Meds and other Supplements

		Calories	Fat grams	Carbs grams	Protein grams	Fiber grams
GRAND TOTALS > DAY#						

Physical Fitness

Type	Hours	Reps/Sets	Intensity	Calories Burned

	Bad									Excellent
My Attitude	1	2	3	4	5	6	7	8	9	10
On Track?	1	2	3	4	5	6	7	8	9	10
Belief Meter	1	2	3	4	5	6	7	8	9	10

_____ _____
Date   Day of the week

Day #

Eat mostly vegetables and fruits.

Breakfast	Quantity	Calories	Fat grams	Carb grams	Protein grams	Fiber grams
Breakfast Totals						

Lunch	Quantity	Calories	Fat grams	Carb grams	Protein grams	Fiber grams
Lunch Totals						

Dinner	Quantity	Calories	Fat grams	Carb grams	Protein grams	Fiber grams
Dinner Totals						

M = Morning
A = Afternoon
E = Evening

Weight

Total 8 oz. glasses of water today:

Snacks	Quantity	Calories	Fat grams	Carbs grams	Protein grams	Fiber grams
Snack Totals						

Vitamins, Meds and other Supplements

		Calories	Fat grams	Carbs grams	Protein grams	Fiber grams
GRAND TOTALS > DAY#						

Physical Fitness

Type	Hours	Reps/Sets	Intensity	Calories Burned

	Bad									Excellent
My Attitude	1	2	3	4	5	6	7	8	9	10
On Track?	1	2	3	4	5	6	7	8	9	10
Belief Meter	1	2	3	4	5	6	7	8	9	10

_____ _____
Date   Day of the week

_____
Day #

Excuses are a practiced form of giving up control to external circumstances and people.

Breakfast	Quantity	Calories	Fat grams	Carb grams	Protein grams	Fiber grams
Breakfast Totals						

Lunch	Quantity	Calories	Fat grams	Carb grams	Protein grams	Fiber grams
Lunch Totals						

Dinner	Quantity	Calories	Fat grams	Carb grams	Protein grams	Fiber grams
Dinner Totals						

Weight

Total 8 oz. glasses of water today:

Snacks	Quantity	Calories	Fat grams	Carbs grams	Protein grams	Fiber grams
Snack Totals						

Vitamins, Meds and other Supplements

		Calories	Fat grams	Carbs grams	Protein grams	Fiber grams
GRAND TOTALS > DAY#						

Physical Fitness

Type	Hours	Reps/Sets	Intensity	Calories Burned

	Bad									Excellent
My Attitude	1	2	3	4	5	6	7	8	9	10
On Track?	1	2	3	4	5	6	7	8	9	10
Belief Meter	1	2	3	4	5	6	7	8	9	10

_____   _____
Date   Day of the week

_____
Day #

Read the nutrition labels and ask restaurants for calorie counts.

Breakfast	Quantity	Calories	Fat grams	Carb grams	Protein grams	Fiber grams
Breakfast Totals						

Lunch	Quantity	Calories	Fat grams	Carb grams	Protein grams	Fiber grams
Lunch Totals						

Dinner	Quantity	Calories	Fat grams	Carb grams	Protein grams	Fiber grams
Dinner Totals						

M = Morning
A = Afternoon
E = Evening

Weight

Total 8 oz. glasses of water today:

Snacks	Quantity	Calories	Fat grams	Carbs grams	Protein grams	Fiber grams
Snack Totals						

Vitamins, Meds and other Supplements

		Calories	Fat grams	Carbs grams	Protein grams	Fiber grams
GRAND TOTALS > DAY#						

Physical Fitness

Type	Hours	Reps/Sets	Intensity	Calories Burned

	Bad									Excellent
My Attitude	1	2	3	4	5	6	7	8	9	10
On Track?	1	2	3	4	5	6	7	8	9	10
Belief Meter	1	2	3	4	5	6	7	8	9	10

_____ Date   _____ Day of the week

_____ Day #

Treat your goals like you have already achieved them and you will.

Breakfast	Quantity	Calories	Fat grams	Carb grams	Protein grams	Fiber grams
Breakfast Totals						
Lunch	Quantity	Calories	Fat grams	Carb grams	Protein grams	Fiber grams
Lunch Totals						
Dinner	Quantity	Calories	Fat grams	Carb grams	Protein grams	Fiber grams
Dinner Totals						

M = Morning
A = Afternoon
E = Evening

Weight

Total 8 oz. glasses of water today:

Snacks	Quantity	Calories	Fat grams	Carbs grams	Protein grams	Fiber grams
Snack Totals						

Vitamins, Meds and other Supplements

	Calories	Fat grams	Carbs grams	Protein grams	Fiber grams
GRAND TOTALS > DAY#					

Physical Fitness

Type	Hours	Reps/Sets	Intensity	Calories Burned

	Bad									Excellent
My Attitude	1	2	3	4	5	6	7	8	9	10
On Track?	1	2	3	4	5	6	7	8	9	10
Belief Meter	1	2	3	4	5	6	7	8	9	10

		Date				Day of the week	

___
Day #

All exercise is cumulative. Just 20 minutes a day equates to more than 121 hours a year.

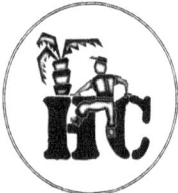

Breakfast	Quantity	Calories	Fat grams	Carb grams	Protein grams	Fiber grams
Breakfast Totals						

Lunch	Quantity	Calories	Fat grams	Carb grams	Protein grams	Fiber grams
Lunch Totals						

Dinner	Quantity	Calories	Fat grams	Carb grams	Protein grams	Fiber grams
Dinner Totals						

Weight

Total 8 oz. glasses
of water today:

Snacks	Quantity	Calories	Fat grams	Carbs grams	Protein grams	Fiber grams
Snack Totals						

Vitamins, Meds and other Supplements

		Calories	Fat grams	Carbs grams	Protein grams	Fiber grams
GRAND TOTALS > DAY#						

Physical Fitness

Type	Hours	Reps/Sets	Intensity	Calories Burned

	Bad									Excellent
My Attitude	1	2	3	4	5	6	7	8	9	10
On Track?	1	2	3	4	5	6	7	8	9	10
Belief Meter	1	2	3	4	5	6	7	8	9	10

_____   _____
Date   Day of the week

Day #

We all need a dose of Vitamin "D," "D" as in discipline.

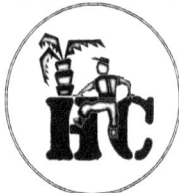

Breakfast	Quantity	Calories	Fat grams	Carb grams	Protein grams	Fiber grams
Breakfast Totals						
Lunch	Quantity	Calories	Fat grams	Carb grams	Protein grams	Fiber grams
Lunch Totals						
Dinner	Quantity	Calories	Fat grams	Carb grams	Protein grams	Fiber grams
Dinner Totals						

M = Morning
A = Afternoon
E = Evening

Weight

Total 8 oz. glasses
of water today:

Snacks	Quantity	Calories	Fat grams	Carbs grams	Protein grams	Fiber grams
Snack Totals						

Vitamins, Meds and other Supplements

		Calories	Fat grams	Carbs grams	Protein grams	Fiber grams
GRAND TOTALS > DAY#						

Physical Fitness

Type	Hours	Reps/Sets	Intensity	Calories Burned

	Bad									Excellent
My Attitude	1	2	3	4	5	6	7	8	9	10
On Track?	1	2	3	4	5	6	7	8	9	10
Belief Meter	1	2	3	4	5	6	7	8	9	10

_____ _____
Date   Day of the week

Day #

You can do it!

Breakfast	Quantity	Calories	Fat grams	Carb grams	Protein grams	Fiber grams
Breakfast Totals						

Lunch	Quantity	Calories	Fat grams	Carb grams	Protein grams	Fiber grams
Lunch Totals						

Dinner	Quantity	Calories	Fat grams	Carb grams	Protein grams	Fiber grams
Dinner Totals						

M = Morning
A = Afternoon
E = Evening

Weight

Total 8 oz. glasses
of water today:

Snacks	Quantity	Calories	Fat grams	Carbs grams	Protein grams	Fiber grams
Snack Totals						

Vitamins, Meds and other Supplements

		Calories	Fat grams	Carbs grams	Protein grams	Fiber grams
GRAND TOTALS > **DAY#**						

Physical Fitness

Type	Hours	Reps/Sets	Intensity	Calories Burned

	Bad									Excellent
My Attitude	1	2	3	4	5	6	7	8	9	10
On Track?	1	2	3	4	5	6	7	8	9	10
Belief Meter	1	2	3	4	5	6	7	8	9	10

_____ _____
Date   Day of the week

_____
Day #

How many times do you get back up when you fall? Every single time!

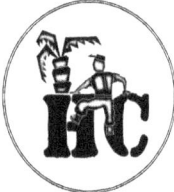

Breakfast	Quantity	Calories	Fat grams	Carb grams	Protein grams	Fiber grams
Breakfast Totals						
Lunch	Quantity	Calories	Fat grams	Carb grams	Protein grams	Fiber grams
Lunch Totals						
Dinner	Quantity	Calories	Fat grams	Carb grams	Protein grams	Fiber grams
Dinner Totals						

M = Morning
A = Afternoon
E = Evening

Weight

Total 8 oz. glasses
of water today:

Snacks	Quantity	Calories	Fat grams	Carbs grams	Protein grams	Fiber grams
Snack Totals						

Vitamins, Meds and other Supplements

		Calories	Fat grams	Carbs grams	Protein grams	Fiber grams
GRAND TOTALS > DAY#						

Physical Fitness

Type	Hours	Reps/Sets	Intensity	Calories Burned

	Bad									Excellent
My Attitude	1	2	3	4	5	6	7	8	9	10
On Track?	1	2	3	4	5	6	7	8	9	10
Belief Meter	1	2	3	4	5	6	7	8	9	10

_____   _____
Date   Day of the week

_____
Day #

Protein does not just run around on two or four legs. Count plant-based protein.

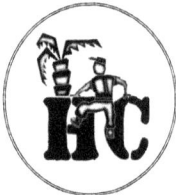

HC

Breakfast	Quantity	Calories	Fat grams	Carb grams	Protein grams	Fiber grams
Breakfast Totals						

Lunch	Quantity	Calories	Fat grams	Carb grams	Protein grams	Fiber grams
Lunch Totals						

Dinner	Quantity	Calories	Fat grams	Carb grams	Protein grams	Fiber grams
Dinner Totals						

M = Morning
A = Afternoon
E = Evening

Weight (   )

Total 8 oz. glasses of water today:

Snacks	Quantity	Calories	Fat grams	Carbs grams	Protein grams	Fiber grams
Snack Totals						

Vitamins, Meds and other Supplements

		Calories	Fat grams	Carbs grams	Protein grams	Fiber grams
GRAND TOTALS > DAY#						

Physical Fitness

Type	Hours	Reps/Sets	Intensity	Calories Burned

	Bad									Excellent
My Attitude	1	2	3	4	5	6	7	8	9	10
On Track?	1	2	3	4	5	6	7	8	9	10
Belief Meter	1	2	3	4	5	6	7	8	9	10

_____ _____
Date   Day of the week

Day #

TV kills, if it's robbing you of heart attack preventing exercise.

Breakfast	Quantity	Calories	Fat grams	Carb grams	Protein grams	Fiber grams
Breakfast Totals						

Lunch	Quantity	Calories	Fat grams	Carb grams	Protein grams	Fiber grams
Lunch Totals						

Dinner	Quantity	Calories	Fat grams	Carb grams	Protein grams	Fiber grams
Dinner Totals						

M = Morning
A = Afternoon
E = Evening

Weight

Total 8 oz. glasses of water today:

Snacks	Quantity	Calories	Fat grams	Carbs grams	Protein grams	Fiber grams
Snack Totals						

Vitamins, Meds and other Supplements

		Calories	Fat grams	Carbs grams	Protein grams	Fiber grams
GRAND TOTALS > DAY#						

Physical Fitness

Type	Hours	Reps/Sets	Intensity	Calories Burned

	Bad									Excellent
My Attitude	1	2	3	4	5	6	7	8	9	10
On Track?	1	2	3	4	5	6	7	8	9	10
Belief Meter	1	2	3	4	5	6	7	8	9	10

_____ _____
Date   Day of the week

Day #

A BMI of 25 or higher is considered overweight.

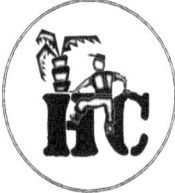

Breakfast	Quantity	Calories	Fat grams	Carb grams	Protein grams	Fiber grams
Breakfast Totals						
Lunch	Quantity	Calories	Fat grams	Carb grams	Protein grams	Fiber grams
Lunch Totals						
Dinner	Quantity	Calories	Fat grams	Carb grams	Protein grams	Fiber grams
Dinner Totals						

M = Morning
A = Afternoon
E = Evening

Weight

Total 8 oz. glasses
of water today:

Snacks	Quantity	Calories	Fat grams	Carbs grams	Protein grams	Fiber grams
Snack Totals						

Vitamins, Meds and other Supplements

		Calories	Fat grams	Carbs grams	Protein grams	Fiber grams
GRAND TOTALS > DAY#						

Physical Fitness

Type	Hours	Reps/Sets	Intensity	Calories Burned

	Bad									Excellent
My Attitude	1	2	3	4	5	6	7	8	9	10
On Track?	1	2	3	4	5	6	7	8	9	10
Belief Meter	1	2	3	4	5	6	7	8	9	10

_____ _____
Date   Day of the week

_____
Day #

Increase your calorie burn. Combine your strength and cardio training.

Breakfast	Quantity	Calories	Fat grams	Carb grams	Protein grams	Fiber grams
Breakfast Totals						

Lunch	Quantity	Calories	Fat grams	Carb grams	Protein grams	Fiber grams
Lunch Totals						

Dinner	Quantity	Calories	Fat grams	Carb grams	Protein grams	Fiber grams
Dinner Totals						

M = Morning
A = Afternoon
E = Evening

Weight

Total 8 oz. glasses of water today:

Snacks	Quantity	Calories	Fat grams	Carbs grams	Protein grams	Fiber grams
Snack Totals						

Vitamins, Meds and other Supplements

		Calories	Fat grams	Carbs grams	Protein grams	Fiber grams
GRAND TOTALS > DAY#						

Physical Fitness

Type	Hours	Reps/Sets	Intensity	Calories Burned

	Bad									Excellent
My Attitude	1	2	3	4	5	6	7	8	9	10
On Track?	1	2	3	4	5	6	7	8	9	10
Belief Meter	1	2	3	4	5	6	7	8	9	10

Date	Day of the week

Day #

Go to the produce section and pick out some healthy snacks of fruits and vegetables.

Breakfast	Quantity	Calories	Fat grams	Carb grams	Protein grams	Fiber grams
Breakfast Totals						

Lunch	Quantity	Calories	Fat grams	Carb grams	Protein grams	Fiber grams
Lunch Totals						

Dinner	Quantity	Calories	Fat grams	Carb grams	Protein grams	Fiber grams
Dinner Totals						

Weight

Total 8 oz. glasses of water today:

Snacks	Quantity	Calories	Fat grams	Carbs grams	Protein grams	Fiber grams
Snack Totals						

Vitamins, Meds and other Supplements

		Calories	Fat grams	Carbs grams	Protein grams	Fiber grams
GRAND TOTALS > DAY#						

Physical Fitness

Type	Hours	Reps/Sets	Intensity	Calories Burned

	Bad									Excellent
My Attitude	1	2	3	4	5	6	7	8	9	10
On Track?	1	2	3	4	5	6	7	8	9	10
Belief Meter	1	2	3	4	5	6	7	8	9	10

_____ _____
Date   Day of the week

Day #

On a scale of 1 to 10 your health is a 10. Live your life accordingly.

Breakfast	Quantity	Calories	Fat grams	Carb grams	Protein grams	Fiber grams
Breakfast Totals						

Lunch	Quantity	Calories	Fat grams	Carb grams	Protein grams	Fiber grams
Lunch Totals						

Dinner	Quantity	Calories	Fat grams	Carb grams	Protein grams	Fiber grams
Dinner Totals						

Weight

Total 8 oz. glasses
of water today:

Snacks	Quantity	Calories	Fat grams	Carbs grams	Protein grams	Fiber grams
Snack Totals						

Vitamins, Meds and other Supplements

		Calories	Fat grams	Carbs grams	Protein grams	Fiber grams
GRAND TOTALS > DAY#						

Physical Fitness

Type	Hours	Reps/Sets	Intensity	Calories Burned

	Bad									Excellent
My Attitude	1	2	3	4	5	6	7	8	9	10
On Track?	1	2	3	4	5	6	7	8	9	10
Belief Meter	1	2	3	4	5	6	7	8	9	10

Day #

Eliminate the flavored beverages and drink water. Result: 100 to 400 calories a day eliminated.

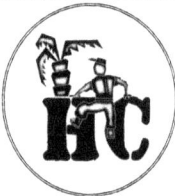

Breakfast	Quantity	Calories	Fat grams	Carb grams	Protein grams	Fiber grams
Breakfast Totals						

Lunch	Quantity	Calories	Fat grams	Carb grams	Protein grams	Fiber grams
Lunch Totals						

Dinner	Quantity	Calories	Fat grams	Carb grams	Protein grams	Fiber grams
Dinner Totals						

M = Morning
A = Afternoon
E = Evening

Weight

Total 8 oz. glasses
of water today:

Snacks	Quantity	Calories	Fat grams	Carbs grams	Protein grams	Fiber grams
Snack Totals						

Vitamins, Meds and other Supplements

		Calories	Fat grams	Carbs grams	Protein grams	Fiber grams
GRAND TOTALS > DAY#						

Physical Fitness

Type	Hours	Reps/Sets	Intensity	Calories Burned

	Bad									Excellent
My Attitude	1	2	3	4	5	6	7	8	9	10
On Track?	1	2	3	4	5	6	7	8	9	10
Belief Meter	1	2	3	4	5	6	7	8	9	10

_____ _____
Date   Day of the week

_____
Day #

Use weight management tools at home: measuring cups, spoons and scales.

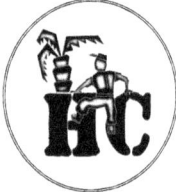

Breakfast	Quantity	Calories	Fat grams	Carb grams	Protein grams	Fiber grams
Breakfast Totals						
Lunch	Quantity	Calories	Fat grams	Carb grams	Protein grams	Fiber grams
Lunch Totals						
Dinner	Quantity	Calories	Fat grams	Carb grams	Protein grams	Fiber grams
Dinner Totals						

M = Morning
A = Afternoon
E = Evening

Weight

Total 8 oz. glasses of water today:

Snacks	Quantity	Calories	Fat grams	Carbs grams	Protein grams	Fiber grams
Snack Totals						

Vitamins, Meds and other Supplements

		Calories	Fat grams	Carbs grams	Protein grams	Fiber grams
GRAND TOTALS > DAY#						

Physical Fitness

Type	Hours	Reps/Sets	Intensity	Calories Burned

	Bad									Excellent
My Attitude	1	2	3	4	5	6	7	8	9	10
On Track?	1	2	3	4	5	6	7	8	9	10
Belief Meter	1	2	3	4	5	6	7	8	9	10

_____
Day #

Weigh yourself regularly and increase your chances of weight loss success by 50 %.

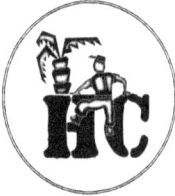

Breakfast	Quantity	Calories	Fat grams	Carb grams	Protein grams	Fiber grams
Breakfast Totals						

Lunch	Quantity	Calories	Fat grams	Carb grams	Protein grams	Fiber grams
Lunch Totals						

Dinner	Quantity	Calories	Fat grams	Carb grams	Protein grams	Fiber grams
Dinner Totals						

Weight

Total 8 oz. glasses of water today:

Snacks	Quantity	Calories	Fat grams	Carbs grams	Protein grams	Fiber grams
Snack Totals						

Vitamins, Meds and other Supplements

		Calories	Fat grams	Carbs grams	Protein grams	Fiber grams
GRAND TOTALS > DAY#						

Physical Fitness

Type	Hours	Reps/Sets	Intensity	Calories Burned

	Bad									Excellent
My Attitude	1	2	3	4	5	6	7	8	9	10
On Track?	1	2	3	4	5	6	7	8	9	10
Belief Meter	1	2	3	4	5	6	7	8	9	10

_____   _____
Date   Day of the week

Day #

Three days of writing down everything you eat and drink with calorie count will cause you to eat less and better.

Breakfast	Quantity	Calories	Fat grams	Carb grams	Protein grams	Fiber grams
Breakfast Totals						

Lunch	Quantity	Calories	Fat grams	Carb grams	Protein grams	Fiber grams
Lunch Totals						

Dinner	Quantity	Calories	Fat grams	Carb grams	Protein grams	Fiber grams
Dinner Totals						

M = Morning
A = Afternoon
E = Evening

Weight ( )

Total 8 oz. glasses of water today:

Snacks	Quantity	Calories	Fat grams	Carbs grams	Protein grams	Fiber grams
Snack Totals						

Vitamins, Meds and other Supplements

	Calories	Fat grams	Carbs grams	Protein grams	Fiber grams
GRAND TOTALS > DAY#					

Physical Fitness

Type	Hours	Reps/Sets	Intensity	Calories Burned

	Bad									Excellent
My Attitude	1	2	3	4	5	6	7	8	9	10
On Track?	1	2	3	4	5	6	7	8	9	10
Belief Meter	1	2	3	4	5	6	7	8	9	10

_____ _____
Date   Day of the week

_____
Day #

Cardio and strength interval training will speed your calorie burn and fitness progress.

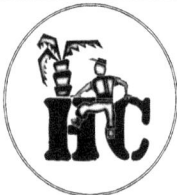

Breakfast	Quantity	Calories	Fat grams	Carb grams	Protein grams	Fiber grams
Breakfast Totals						
Lunch	Quantity	Calories	Fat grams	Carb grams	Protein grams	Fiber grams
Lunch Totals						
Dinner	Quantity	Calories	Fat grams	Carb grams	Protein grams	Fiber grams
Dinner Totals						

M = Morning
A = Afternoon
E = Evening

Weight

Total 8 oz. glasses
of water today:

Snacks	Quantity	Calories	Fat grams	Carbs grams	Protein grams	Fiber grams
Snack Totals						

Vitamins, Meds and other Supplements

		Calories	Fat grams	Carbs grams	Protein grams	Fiber grams
GRAND TOTALS > DAY#						

Physical Fitness

Type	Hours	Reps/Sets	Intensity	Calories Burned

	Poor									Excellent
My Attitude	1	2	3	4	5	6	7	8	9	10
On Track?	1	2	3	4	5	6	7	8	9	10
Belief Meter	1	2	3	4	5	6	7	8	9	10

Day # _____

Two tablespoons of peanut butter equals 188 calories, level tablespoons not heaping.

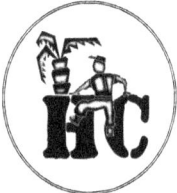

Breakfast	Quantity	Calories	Fat grams	Carb grams	Protein grams	Fiber grams
Breakfast Totals						

Lunch	Quantity	Calories	Fat grams	Carb grams	Protein grams	Fiber grams
Lunch Totals						

Dinner	Quantity	Calories	Fat grams	Carb grams	Protein grams	Fiber grams
Dinner Totals						

M = Morning
A = Afternoon
E = Evening

Weight

Total 8 oz. glasses of water today:

Snacks	Quantity	Calories	Fat grams	Carbs grams	Protein grams	Fiber grams
Snack Totals						

Vitamins, Meds and other Supplements

		Calories	Fat grams	Carbs grams	Protein grams	Fiber grams
GRAND TOTALS > DAY#						

Physical Fitness

Type	Hours	Reps/Sets	Intensity	Calories Burned

	Bad									Excellent
My Attitude	1	2	3	4	5	6	7	8	9	10
On Track?	1	2	3	4	5	6	7	8	9	10
Belief Meter	1	2	3	4	5	6	7	8	9	10

_____
Day #

When eating out, plan in advance how you will eat to keep the calories under control.

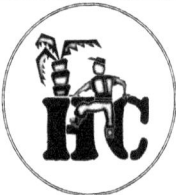

Breakfast	Quantity	Calories	Fat grams	Carb grams	Protein grams	Fiber grams
Breakfast Totals						

Lunch	Quantity	Calories	Fat grams	Carb grams	Protein grams	Fiber grams
Lunch Totals						

Dinner	Quantity	Calories	Fat grams	Carb grams	Protein grams	Fiber grams
Dinner Totals						

M = Morning
A = Afternoon
E = Evening

Weight

Total 8 oz. glasses of water today:

Snacks	Quantity	Calories	Fat grams	Carbs grams	Protein grams	Fiber grams
Snack Totals						

Vitamins, Meds and other Supplements

		Calories	Fat grams	Carbs grams	Protein grams	Fiber grams
GRAND TOTALS > **DAY#**						

Physical Fitness

Type	Hours	Reps/Sets	Intensity	Calories Burned

	Bad									Excellent
My Attitude	1	2	3	4	5	6	7	8	9	10
On Track?	1	2	3	4	5	6	7	8	9	10
Belief Meter	1	2	3	4	5	6	7	8	9	10

_____ _____
Date   Day of the week

Day #

Treat yourself once a week to whatever you like to eat.

Breakfast	Quantity	Calories	Fat grams	Carb grams	Protein grams	Fiber grams
Breakfast Totals						

Lunch	Quantity	Calories	Fat grams	Carb grams	Protein grams	Fiber grams
Lunch Totals						

Dinner	Quantity	Calories	Fat grams	Carb grams	Protein grams	Fiber grams
Dinner Totals						

M = Morning
A = Afternoon
E = Evening

Weight

Total 8 oz. glasses of water today:

Snacks	Quantity	Calories	Fat grams	Carbs grams	Protein grams	Fiber grams
Snack Totals						

Vitamins, Meds and other Supplements

		Calories	Fat grams	Carbs grams	Protein grams	Fiber grams
GRAND TOTALS > DAY#						

Physical Fitness

Type	Hours	Reps/Sets	Intensity	Calories Burned

	Bad									Excellent
My Attitude	1	2	3	4	5	6	7	8	9	10
On Track?	1	2	3	4	5	6	7	8	9	10
Belief Meter	1	2	3	4	5	6	7	8	9	10

Day #

Negative emotions of anger, bitterness or frustration can cause overindulgence and health problems.

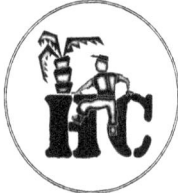

Breakfast	Quantity	Calories	Fat grams	Carb grams	Protein grams	Fiber grams
Breakfast Totals						

Lunch	Quantity	Calories	Fat grams	Carb grams	Protein grams	Fiber grams
Lunch Totals						

Dinner	Quantity	Calories	Fat grams	Carb grams	Protein grams	Fiber grams
Dinner Totals						

M = Morning
A = Afternoon
E = Evening

Weight

Total 8 oz. glasses
of water today:

Snacks	Quantity	Calories	Fat grams	Carbs grams	Protein grams	Fiber grams
Snack Totals						

Vitamins, Meds and other Supplements

		Calories	Fat grams	Carbs grams	Protein grams	Fiber grams
GRAND TOTALS > DAY#						

Physical Fitness

Type	Hours	Reps/Sets	Intensity	Calories Burned

	Bad									Excellent
My Attitude	1	2	3	4	5	6	7	8	9	10
On Track?	1	2	3	4	5	6	7	8	9	10
Belief Meter	1	2	3	4	5	6	7	8	9	10

_____
Day #

Seek first what you need and you'll find that it's what you want.

Breakfast	Quantity	Calories	Fat grams	Carb grams	Protein grams	Fiber grams
Breakfast Totals						

Lunch	Quantity	Calories	Fat grams	Carb grams	Protein grams	Fiber grams
Lunch Totals						

Dinner	Quantity	Calories	Fat grams	Carb grams	Protein grams	Fiber grams
Dinner Totals						

M = Morning
A = Afternoon
E = Evening

Weight

Total 8 oz. glasses
of water today:

Snacks	Quantity	Calories	Fat grams	Carbs grams	Protein grams	Fiber grams
Snack Totals						

Vitamins, Meds and other Supplements

		Calories	Fat grams	Carbs grams	Protein grams	Fiber grams
GRAND TOTALS > DAY#						

Physical Fitness

Type	Hours	Reps/Sets	Intensity	Calories Burned

	Bad									Excellent
My Attitude	1	2	3	4	5	6	7	8	9	10
On Track?	1	2	3	4	5	6	7	8	9	10
Belief Meter	1	2	3	4	5	6	7	8	9	10

_____
Day #

Delayed gratification rewards you with what you really need.

Breakfast	Quantity	Calories	Fat grams	Carb grams	Protein grams	Fiber grams
Breakfast Totals						
Lunch	Quantity	Calories	Fat grams	Carb grams	Protein grams	Fiber grams
Lunch Totals						
Dinner	Quantity	Calories	Fat grams	Carb grams	Protein grams	Fiber grams
Dinner Totals						

M = Morning
A = Afternoon
E = Evening

Weight

Total 8 oz. glasses of water today:

Snacks	Quantity	Calories	Fat grams	Carbs grams	Protein grams	Fiber grams
Snack Totals						

Vitamins, Meds and other Supplements

		Calories	Fat grams	Carbs grams	Protein grams	Fiber grams
GRAND TOTALS > DAY#						

Physical Fitness

Type	Hours	Reps/Sets	Intensity	Calories Burned

	Bad									Excellent
My Attitude	1	2	3	4	5	6	7	8	9	10
On Track?	1	2	3	4	5	6	7	8	9	10
Belief Meter	1	2	3	4	5	6	7	8	9	10

_____ _____
Date   Day of the week

Day #

3,500 calories equals one pound of body fat.

Breakfast	Quantity	Calories	Fat grams	Carb grams	Protein grams	Fiber grams
Breakfast Totals						

Lunch	Quantity	Calories	Fat grams	Carb grams	Protein grams	Fiber grams
Lunch Totals						

Dinner	Quantity	Calories	Fat grams	Carb grams	Protein grams	Fiber grams
Dinner Totals						

M = Morning
A = Afternoon
E = Evening

Weight ⬭

Total 8 oz. glasses of water today:

Snacks	Quantity	Calories	Fat grams	Carbs grams	Protein grams	Fiber grams
Snack Totals						

Vitamins, Meds and other Supplements

		Calories	Fat grams	Carbs grams	Protein grams	Fiber grams
GRAND TOTALS > DAY#						

Physical Fitness

Type	Hours	Reps/Sets	Intensity	Calories Burned

	Bad									Excellent
My Attitude	1	2	3	4	5	6	7	8	9	10
On Track?	1	2	3	4	5	6	7	8	9	10
Belief Meter	1	2	3	4	5	6	7	8	9	10

Date _____   Day of the week _____

___
Day #

Use the 15/30/55 rule when eating. 15 % protein, 30 % fat and 55 % carbohydrates.

Breakfast	Quantity	Calories	Fat grams	Carb grams	Protein grams	Fiber grams
Breakfast Totals						

Lunch	Quantity	Calories	Fat grams	Carb grams	Protein grams	Fiber grams
Lunch Totals						

Dinner	Quantity	Calories	Fat grams	Carb grams	Protein grams	Fiber grams
Dinner Totals						

M = Morning
A = Afternoon
E = Evening

Weight

Total 8 oz. glasses
of water today:

Snacks	Quantity	Calories	Fat grams	Carbs grams	Protein grams	Fiber grams
Snack Totals						

Vitamins, Meds and other Supplements

		Calories	Fat grams	Carbs grams	Protein grams	Fiber grams
GRAND TOTALS > **DAY#**						

Physical Fitness

Type	Hours	Reps/Sets	Intensity	Calories Burned

	Bad									Excellent
My Attitude	1	2	3	4	5	6	7	8	9	10
On Track?	1	2	3	4	5	6	7	8	9	10
Belief Meter	1	2	3	4	5	6	7	8	9	10

_____
Date

_____
Day of the week

_____
Day #

Fifty percent of those overweight do not eat breakfast.

Breakfast	Quantity	Calories	Fat grams	Carb grams	Protein grams	Fiber grams
Breakfast Totals						

Lunch	Quantity	Calories	Fat grams	Carb grams	Protein grams	Fiber grams
Lunch Totals						

Dinner	Quantity	Calories	Fat grams	Carb grams	Protein grams	Fiber grams
Dinner Totals						

M = Morning
A = Afternoon
E = Evening

Weight

Total 8 oz. glasses
of water today:

Snacks	Quantity	Calories	Fat grams	Carbs grams	Protein grams	Fiber grams
Snack Totals						

Vitamins, Meds and other Supplements

		Calories	Fat grams	Carbs grams	Protein grams	Fiber grams
GRAND TOTALS > DAY#						

Physical Fitness

Type	Hours	Reps/Sets	Intensity	Calories Burned

	Bad									Excellent
My Attitude	1	2	3	4	5	6	7	8	9	10
On Track?	1	2	3	4	5	6	7	8	9	10
Belief Meter	1	2	3	4	5	6	7	8	9	10

_____   _____
Date   Day of the week

Day #

Be aware of quantity and quality of foods you eat.

Breakfast	Quantity	Calories	Fat grams	Carb grams	Protein grams	Fiber grams
Breakfast Totals						

Lunch	Quantity	Calories	Fat grams	Carb grams	Protein grams	Fiber grams
Lunch Totals						

Dinner	Quantity	Calories	Fat grams	Carb grams	Protein grams	Fiber grams
Dinner Totals						

M = Morning
A = Afternoon
E = Evening

Weight

Total 8 oz. glasses
of water today:

Snacks	Quantity	Calories	Fat grams	Carbs grams	Protein grams	Fiber grams
Snack Totals						

Vitamins, Meds and other Supplements

		Calories	Fat grams	Carbs grams	Protein grams	Fiber grams
GRAND TOTALS > DAY#						

Physical Fitness

Type	Hours	Reps/Sets	Intensity	Calories Burned

	Bad									Excellent
My Attitude	1	2	3	4	5	6	7	8	9	10
On Track?	1	2	3	4	5	6	7	8	9	10
Belief Meter	1	2	3	4	5	6	7	8	9	10

_____ Date   _____ Day of the week

_____
Day #

Make all your decisions based on the long-term impact.

Breakfast	Quantity	Calories	Fat grams	Carb grams	Protein grams	Fiber grams
Breakfast Totals						
Lunch	Quantity	Calories	Fat grams	Carb grams	Protein grams	Fiber grams
Lunch Totals						
Dinner	Quantity	Calories	Fat grams	Carb grams	Protein grams	Fiber grams
Dinner Totals						

M = Morning
A = Afternoon
E = Evening

Weight

Total 8 oz. glasses
of water today:

Snacks	Quantity	Calories	Fat grams	Carbs grams	Protein grams	Fiber grams
Snack Totals						

Vitamins, Meds and other Supplements

		Calories	Fat grams	Carbs grams	Protein grams	Fiber grams
GRAND TOTALS > DAY#						

Physical Fitness

Type	Hours	Reps/Sets	Intensity	Calories Burned

	Bad									Excellent
My Attitude	1	2	3	4	5	6	7	8	9	10
On Track?	1	2	3	4	5	6	7	8	9	10
Belief Meter	1	2	3	4	5	6	7	8	9	10

_____ _____
Date   Day of the week

_____ **Day #**

Make all your decisions based on what is most important for you and those around you.

Breakfast	Quantity	Calories	Fat grams	Carb grams	Protein grams	Fiber grams
Breakfast Totals						
Lunch	Quantity	Calories	Fat grams	Carb grams	Protein grams	Fiber grams
Lunch Totals						
Dinner	Quantity	Calories	Fat grams	Carb grams	Protein grams	Fiber grams
Dinner Totals						

Weight

Total 8 oz. glasses
of water today:

Snacks	Quantity	Calories	Fat grams	Carbs grams	Protein grams	Fiber grams
Snack Totals						

Vitamins, Meds and other Supplements

		Calories	Fat grams	Carbs grams	Protein grams	Fiber grams
GRAND TOTALS > DAY#						

Physical Fitness

Type	Hours	Reps/Sets	Intensity	Calories Burned

	Bad									Excellent
My Attitude	1	2	3	4	5	6	7	8	9	10
On Track?	1	2	3	4	5	6	7	8	9	10
Belief Meter	1	2	3	4	5	6	7	8	9	10

_____ _____
Date   Day of the week

Day #

Eat three meals and two healthy snacks a day.

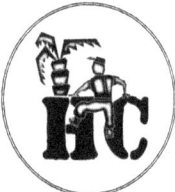

Breakfast	Quantity	Calories	Fat grams	Carb grams	Protein grams	Fiber grams
Breakfast Totals						
Lunch	Quantity	Calories	Fat grams	Carb grams	Protein grams	Fiber grams
Lunch Totals						
Dinner	Quantity	Calories	Fat grams	Carb grams	Protein grams	Fiber grams
Dinner Totals						

M = Morning
A = Afternoon
E = Evening

Weight

Total 8 oz. glasses
of water today:

Snacks	Quantity	Calories	Fat grams	Carbs grams	Protein grams	Fiber grams
Snack Totals						

Vitamins, Meds and other Supplements

		Calories	Fat grams	Carbs grams	Protein grams	Fiber grams
GRAND TOTALS > DAY#						

Physical Fitness

Type	Hours	Reps/Sets	Intensity	Calories Burned

	Bad									Excellent
My Attitude	1	2	3	4	5	6	7	8	9	10
On Track?	1	2	3	4	5	6	7	8	9	10
Belief Meter	1	2	3	4	5	6	7	8	9	10

| | | Date | | | | | | Day of the week |

Day #

We are eating 300
calories a day more than
Americans 30 years ago.
That's 109,500 calories a
year.

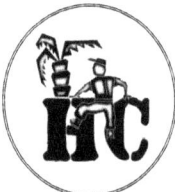

Breakfast	Quantity	Calories	Fat grams	Carb grams	Protein grams	Fiber grams
Breakfast Totals						

Lunch	Quantity	Calories	Fat grams	Carb grams	Protein grams	Fiber grams
Lunch Totals						

Dinner	Quantity	Calories	Fat grams	Carb grams	Protein grams	Fiber grams
Dinner Totals						

Weight

Total 8 oz. glasses of water today:

Snacks	Quantity	Calories	Fat grams	Carbs grams	Protein grams	Fiber grams
Snack Totals						

Vitamins, Meds and other Supplements

		Calories	Fat grams	Carbs grams	Protein grams	Fiber grams
GRAND TOTALS > DAY#						

Physical Fitness

Type	Hours	Reps/Sets	Intensity	Calories Burned

	Bad									Excellent
My Attitude	1	2	3	4	5	6	7	8	9	10
On Track?	1	2	3	4	5	6	7	8	9	10
Belief Meter	1	2	3	4	5	6	7	8	9	10

Day #

One in five children in the U.S. are overweight.

Breakfast	Quantity	Calories	Fat grams	Carb grams	Protein grams	Fiber grams
Breakfast Totals						

Lunch	Quantity	Calories	Fat grams	Carb grams	Protein grams	Fiber grams
Lunch Totals						

Dinner	Quantity	Calories	Fat grams	Carb grams	Protein grams	Fiber grams
Dinner Totals						

M = Morning
A = Afternoon
E = Evening

Weight

Total 8 oz. glasses of water today:

Snacks	Quantity	Calories	Fat grams	Carbs grams	Protein grams	Fiber grams
Snack Totals						

Vitamins, Meds and other Supplements

		Calories	Fat grams	Carbs grams	Protein grams	Fiber grams
GRAND TOTALS > DAY#						

Physical Fitness

Type	Hours	Reps/Sets	Intensity	Calories Burned

	Bad									Excellent
My Attitude	1	2	3	4	5	6	7	8	9	10
On Track?	1	2	3	4	5	6	7	8	9	10
Belief Meter	1	2	3	4	5	6	7	8	9	10

_____ _____
Date   Day of the week

_____
Day #

Do at least five sets of push-ups a day.

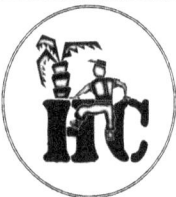

Breakfast	Quantity	Calories	Fat grams	Carb grams	Protein grams	Fiber grams
Breakfast Totals						

Lunch	Quantity	Calories	Fat grams	Carb grams	Protein grams	Fiber grams
Lunch Totals						

Dinner	Quantity	Calories	Fat grams	Carb grams	Protein grams	Fiber grams
Dinner Totals						

M = Morning
A = Afternoon
E = Evening

Weight

Total 8 oz. glasses of water today:

Snacks	Quantity	Calories	Fat grams	Carbs grams	Protein grams	Fiber grams
Snack Totals						

Vitamins, Meds and other Supplements

		Calories	Fat grams	Carbs grams	Protein grams	Fiber grams
GRAND TOTALS > DAY#						

Physical Fitness

Type	Hours	Reps/Sets	Intensity	Calories Burned

	Bad									Excellent
My Attitude	1	2	3	4	5	6	7	8	9	10
On Track?	1	2	3	4	5	6	7	8	9	10
Belief Meter	1	2	3	4	5	6	7	8	9	10

_____ Date   _____ Day of the week

_____
Day #

Do at least 100 crunches a day.

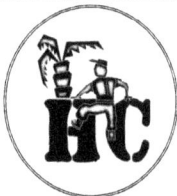

Breakfast	Quantity	Calories	Fat grams	Carb grams	Protein grams	Fiber grams
Breakfast Totals						
Lunch	Quantity	Calories	Fat grams	Carb grams	Protein grams	Fiber grams
Lunch Totals						
Dinner	Quantity	Calories	Fat grams	Carb grams	Protein grams	Fiber grams
Dinner Totals						

Weight

Total 8 oz. glasses of water today:

Snacks	Quantity	Calories	Fat grams	Carbs grams	Protein grams	Fiber grams
Snack Totals						

Vitamins, Meds and other Supplements

		Calories	Fat grams	Carbs grams	Protein grams	Fiber grams
GRAND TOTALS > DAY#						

Physical Fitness

Type	Hours	Reps/Sets	Intensity	Calories Burned

	Bad									Excellent
My Attitude	1	2	3	4	5	6	7	8	9	10
On Track?	1	2	3	4	5	6	7	8	9	10
Belief Meter	1	2	3	4	5	6	7	8	9	10

_____
Day #

Find out what God likes and then do it.

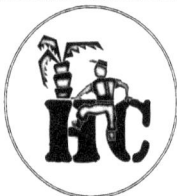

Breakfast	Quantity	Calories	Fat grams	Carb grams	Protein grams	Fiber grams
Breakfast Totals						
Lunch	Quantity	Calories	Fat grams	Carb grams	Protein grams	Fiber grams
Lunch Totals						
Dinner	Quantity	Calories	Fat grams	Carb grams	Protein grams	Fiber grams
Dinner Totals						

Weight

Total 8 oz. glasses
of water today:

Snacks	Quantity	Calories	Fat grams	Carbs grams	Protein grams	Fiber grams
Snack Totals						

Vitamins, Meds and other Supplements

		Calories	Fat grams	Carbs grams	Protein grams	Fiber grams
GRAND TOTALS > **DAY#**						

Physical Fitness

Type	Hours	Reps/Sets	Intensity	Calories Burned

	Bad									Excellent
My Attitude	1	2	3	4	5	6	7	8	9	10
On Track?	1	2	3	4	5	6	7	8	9	10
Belief Meter	1	2	3	4	5	6	7	8	9	10

_____ _____
Date   Day of the week

_____
Day #

All lack of exercise is cumulative. Every hour per day you don't exercise equates to 365 hours a year.

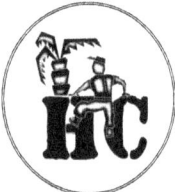

Breakfast	Quantity	Calories	Fat grams	Carb grams	Protein grams	Fiber grams
Breakfast Totals						
Lunch	Quantity	Calories	Fat grams	Carb grams	Protein grams	Fiber grams
Lunch Totals						
Dinner	Quantity	Calories	Fat grams	Carb grams	Protein grams	Fiber grams
Dinner Totals						

M = Morning
A = Afternoon
E = Evening

Weight

Total 8 oz. glasses
of water today:

Snacks	Quantity	Calories	Fat grams	Carbs grams	Protein grams	Fiber grams
Snack Totals						

Vitamins, Meds and other Supplements

		Calories	Fat grams	Carbs grams	Protein grams	Fiber grams
GRAND TOTALS > DAY#						

Physical Fitness

Type	Hours	Reps/Sets	Intensity	Calories Burned

	Bad									Excellent
My Attitude	1	2	3	4	5	6	7	8	9	10
On Track?	1	2	3	4	5	6	7	8	9	10
Belief Meter	1	2	3	4	5	6	7	8	9	10

_____   _____
Date   Day of the week

(_____ Day #)

We were born to do push-ups. It's one of the first moves a baby makes.

Breakfast	Quantity	Calories	Fat grams	Carb grams	Protein grams	Fiber grams
Breakfast Totals						
Lunch	Quantity	Calories	Fat grams	Carb grams	Protein grams	Fiber grams
Lunch Totals						
Dinner	Quantity	Calories	Fat grams	Carb grams	Protein grams	Fiber grams
Dinner Totals						

M = Morning
A = Afternoon
E = Evening

Weight

Total 8 oz. glasses of water today:

Snacks	Quantity	Calories	Fat grams	Carbs grams	Protein grams	Fiber grams
Snack Totals						

Vitamins, Meds and other Supplements

		Calories	Fat grams	Carbs grams	Protein grams	Fiber grams
GRAND TOTALS > DAY#						

Physical Fitness

Type	Hours	Reps/Sets	Intensity	Calories Burned

	Bad									Excellent
My Attitude	1	2	3	4	5	6	7	8	9	10
On Track?	1	2	3	4	5	6	7	8	9	10
Belief Meter	1	2	3	4	5	6	7	8	9	10

_____ _____
Date   Day of the week

Day # _____

Overcome all obstacles.

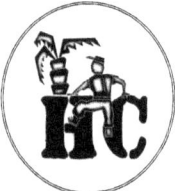

Breakfast	Quantity	Calories	Fat grams	Carb grams	Protein grams	Fiber grams
Breakfast Totals						

Lunch	Quantity	Calories	Fat grams	Carb grams	Protein grams	Fiber grams
Lunch Totals						

Dinner	Quantity	Calories	Fat grams	Carb grams	Protein grams	Fiber grams
Dinner Totals						

	Weight			Total 8 oz. glasses of water today:			

M = Morning
A = Afternoon
E = Evening

Snacks	Quantity	Calories	Fat grams	Carbs grams	Protein grams	Fiber grams
Snack Totals						

Vitamins, Meds and other Supplements

		Calories	Fat grams	Carbs grams	Protein grams	Fiber grams
GRAND TOTALS > DAY#						

Physical Fitness

Type	Hours	Reps/Sets	Intensity	Calories Burned

My Attitude	Bad 1	2	3	4	5	6	7	8	9	Excellent 10
On Track?	1	2	3	4	5	6	7	8	9	10
Belief Meter	1	2	3	4	5	6	7	8	9	10

___
Day #

Be kind to everyone you meet.

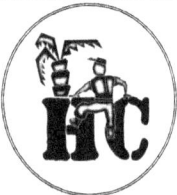

Breakfast	Quantity	Calories	Fat grams	Carb grams	Protein grams	Fiber grams
Breakfast Totals						

Lunch	Quantity	Calories	Fat grams	Carb grams	Protein grams	Fiber grams
Lunch Totals						

Dinner	Quantity	Calories	Fat grams	Carb grams	Protein grams	Fiber grams
Dinner Totals						

M = Morning
A = Afternoon
E = Evening

Weight

Total 8 oz. glasses of water today:

Snacks	Quantity	Calories	Fat grams	Carbs grams	Protein grams	Fiber grams
Snack Totals						

Vitamins, Meds and other Supplements

		Calories	Fat grams	Carbs grams	Protein grams	Fiber grams
GRAND TOTALS > **DAY#**						

Physical Fitness

Type	Hours	Reps/Sets	Intensity	Calories Burned

	Bad									Excellent
My Attitude	1	2	3	4	5	6	7	8	9	10
On Track?	1	2	3	4	5	6	7	8	9	10
Belief Meter	1	2	3	4	5	6	7	8	9	10

Date

Day of the week

Day #

Treat yourself as you would a very best friend.

Breakfast	Quantity	Calories	Fat grams	Carb grams	Protein grams	Fiber grams
Breakfast Totals						

Lunch	Quantity	Calories	Fat grams	Carb grams	Protein grams	Fiber grams
Lunch Totals						

Dinner	Quantity	Calories	Fat grams	Carb grams	Protein grams	Fiber grams
Dinner Totals						

Weight

Total 8 oz. glasses
of water today:

Snacks	Quantity	Calories	Fat grams	Carbs grams	Protein grams	Fiber grams
Snack Totals						

Vitamins, Meds and other Supplements

		Calories	Fat grams	Carbs grams	Protein grams	Fiber grams
GRAND TOTALS > DAY#						

Physical Fitness

Type	Hours	Reps/Sets	Intensity	Calories Burned

	Bad									Excellent
My Attitude	1	2	3	4	5	6	7	8	9	10
On Track?	1	2	3	4	5	6	7	8	9	10
Belief Meter	1	2	3	4	5	6	7	8	9	10

| | Date | | Day of the week |

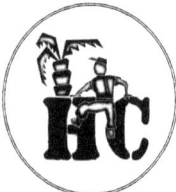

Day #

Give yourself permission to make mistakes and learn from them.

Breakfast	Quantity	Calories	Fat grams	Carb grams	Protein grams	Fiber grams
Breakfast Totals						
Lunch	Quantity	Calories	Fat grams	Carb grams	Protein grams	Fiber grams
Lunch Totals						
Dinner	Quantity	Calories	Fat grams	Carb grams	Protein grams	Fiber grams
Dinner Totals						

Weight

Total 8 oz. glasses of water today:

Snacks	Quantity	Calories	Fat grams	Carbs grams	Protein grams	Fiber grams
Snack Totals						

Vitamins, Meds and other Supplements

		Calories	Fat grams	Carbs grams	Protein grams	Fiber grams
GRAND TOTALS > DAY#						

Physical Fitness

Type	Hours	Reps/Sets	Intensity	Calories Burned

	Bad									Excellent
My Attitude	1	2	3	4	5	6	7	8	9	10
On Track?	1	2	3	4	5	6	7	8	9	10
Belief Meter	1	2	3	4	5	6	7	8	9	10

_____ Date   _____ Day of the week

_____
Day #

Drink 8 to 10 glasses of water a day, more if you are working in heat and humidity.

Breakfast	Quantity	Calories	Fat grams	Carb grams	Protein grams	Fiber grams
Breakfast Totals						
Lunch	Quantity	Calories	Fat grams	Carb grams	Protein grams	Fiber grams
Lunch Totals						
Dinner	Quantity	Calories	Fat grams	Carb grams	Protein grams	Fiber grams
Dinner Totals						

M = Morning
A = Afternoon
E = Evening

Weight

Total 8 oz. glasses
of water today:

Snacks	Quantity	Calories	Fat grams	Carbs grams	Protein grams	Fiber grams
Snack Totals						

Vitamins, Meds and other Supplements

		Calories	Fat grams	Carbs grams	Protein grams	Fiber grams
GRAND TOTALS > DAY#						

Physical Fitness

Type	Hours	Reps/Sets	Intensity	Calories Burned

	Bad									Excellent
My Attitude	1	2	3	4	5	6	7	8	9	10
On Track?	1	2	3	4	5	6	7	8	9	10
Belief Meter	1	2	3	4	5	6	7	8	9	10

_____
Day #

Always listen to your body when training.

Breakfast	Quantity	Calories	Fat grams	Carb grams	Protein grams	Fiber grams
Breakfast Totals						

Lunch	Quantity	Calories	Fat grams	Carb grams	Protein grams	Fiber grams
Lunch Totals						

Dinner	Quantity	Calories	Fat grams	Carb grams	Protein grams	Fiber grams
Dinner Totals						

M = Morning
A = Afternoon
E = Evening

Weight

Total 8 oz. glasses
of water today:

Snacks	Quantity	Calories	Fat grams	Carbs grams	Protein grams	Fiber grams
Snack Totals						

Vitamins, Meds and other Supplements

		Calories	Fat grams	Carbs grams	Protein grams	Fiber grams
GRAND TOTALS > DAY#						

Physical Fitness

Type	Hours	Reps/Sets	Intensity	Calories Burned

	Bad									Excellent
My Attitude	1	2	3	4	5	6	7	8	9	10
On Track?	1	2	3	4	5	6	7	8	9	10
Belief Meter	1	2	3	4	5	6	7	8	9	10

_____ Date _____ Day of the week

_____ Day #

You must meet my friend fatigue before you can meet my friend progress.

Breakfast	Quantity	Calories	Fat grams	Carb grams	Protein grams	Fiber grams
Breakfast Totals						

Lunch	Quantity	Calories	Fat grams	Carb grams	Protein grams	Fiber grams
Lunch Totals						

Dinner	Quantity	Calories	Fat grams	Carb grams	Protein grams	Fiber grams
Dinner Totals						

M = Morning
A = Afternoon
E = Evening

Weight

Total 8 oz. glasses of water today:

Snacks	Quantity	Calories	Fat grams	Carbs grams	Protein grams	Fiber grams
Snack Totals						

Vitamins, Meds and other Supplements

		Calories	Fat grams	Carbs grams	Protein grams	Fiber grams
GRAND TOTALS > DAY#						

Physical Fitness

Type	Hours	Reps/Sets	Intensity	Calories Burned

	Bad									Excellent
My Attitude	1	2	3	4	5	6	7	8	9	10
On Track?	1	2	3	4	5	6	7	8	9	10
Belief Meter	1	2	3	4	5	6	7	8	9	10

_____
Day #

I am alive and
thankful! Today is a
great day to be
alive.

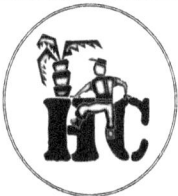

Breakfast	Quantity	Calories	Fat grams	Carb grams	Protein grams	Fiber grams
Breakfast Totals						
Lunch	Quantity	Calories	Fat grams	Carb grams	Protein grams	Fiber grams
Lunch Totals						
Dinner	Quantity	Calories	Fat grams	Carb grams	Protein grams	Fiber grams
Dinner Totals						

Weight

Total 8 oz. glasses of water today:

Snacks	Quantity	Calories	Fat grams	Carbs grams	Protein grams	Fiber grams
Snack Totals						

Vitamins, Meds and other Supplements

		Calories	Fat grams	Carbs grams	Protein grams	Fiber grams
GRAND TOTALS > DAY#						

Physical Fitness

Type	Hours	Reps/Sets	Intensity	Calories Burned

	Bad									Excellent
My Attitude	1	2	3	4	5	6	7	8	9	10
On Track?	1	2	3	4	5	6	7	8	9	10
Belief Meter	1	2	3	4	5	6	7	8	9	10

_____   _____
Date   Day of the week

Day #

I will help as
many people
as I can today.

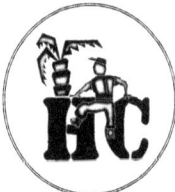

Breakfast	Quantity	Calories	Fat grams	Carb grams	Protein grams	Fiber grams
Breakfast Totals						

Lunch	Quantity	Calories	Fat grams	Carb grams	Protein grams	Fiber grams
Lunch Totals						

Dinner	Quantity	Calories	Fat grams	Carb grams	Protein grams	Fiber grams
Dinner Totals						

M = Morning
A = Afternoon
E = Evening

Weight

Total 8 oz. glasses
of water today:

Snacks	Quantity	Calories	Fat grams	Carbs grams	Protein grams	Fiber grams
Snack Totals						

Vitamins, Meds and other Supplements

		Calories	Fat grams	Carbs grams	Protein grams	Fiber grams
GRAND TOTALS > **DAY#**						

Physical Fitness

Type	Hours	Reps/Sets	Intensity	Calories Burned

	Bad									Excellent
My Attitude	1	2	3	4	5	6	7	8	9	10
On Track?	1	2	3	4	5	6	7	8	9	10
Belief Meter	1	2	3	4	5	6	7	8	9	10

_____
Day #

I will be a role model in all that I say and do.

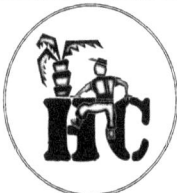

Breakfast	Quantity	Calories	Fat grams	Carb grams	Protein grams	Fiber grams
Breakfast Totals						

Lunch	Quantity	Calories	Fat grams	Carb grams	Protein grams	Fiber grams
Lunch Totals						

Dinner	Quantity	Calories	Fat grams	Carb grams	Protein grams	Fiber grams
Dinner Totals						

M = Morning
A = Afternoon
E = Evening

Weight

Total 8 oz. glasses
of water today:

Snacks	Quantity	Calories	Fat grams	Carbs grams	Protein grams	Fiber grams
Snack Totals						

Vitamins, Meds and other Supplements

		Calories	Fat grams	Carbs grams	Protein grams	Fiber grams
GRAND TOTALS > DAY#						

Physical Fitness

Type	Hours	Reps/Sets	Intensity	Calories Burned

	Bad									Excellent
My Attitude	1	2	3	4	5	6	7	8	9	10
On Track?	1	2	3	4	5	6	7	8	9	10
Belief Meter	1	2	3	4	5	6	7	8	9	10

_____ _____
Date   Day of the week

Day #

Get at least 30 to 40 grams of fiber a day from the food you eat.

Breakfast	Quantity	Calories	Fat grams	Carb grams	Protein grams	Fiber grams
Breakfast Totals						
Lunch	Quantity	Calories	Fat grams	Carb grams	Protein grams	Fiber grams
Lunch Totals						
Dinner	Quantity	Calories	Fat grams	Carb grams	Protein grams	Fiber grams
Dinner Totals						

Weight

Total 8 oz. glasses
of water today:

Snacks	Quantity	Calories	Fat grams	Carbs grams	Protein grams	Fiber grams
Snack Totals						

Vitamins, Meds and other Supplements

		Calories	Fat grams	Carbs grams	Protein grams	Fiber grams
GRAND TOTALS > DAY#						

Physical Fitness

Type	Hours	Reps/Sets	Intensity	Calories Burned

	Bad									Excellent
My Attitude	1	2	3	4	5	6	7	8	9	10
On Track?	1	2	3	4	5	6	7	8	9	10
Belief Meter	1	2	3	4	5	6	7	8	9	10

_____ Date   _____ Day of the week

Day #

Eat fish twice a week.

Breakfast	Quantity	Calories	Fat grams	Carb grams	Protein grams	Fiber grams
Breakfast Totals						

Lunch	Quantity	Calories	Fat grams	Carb grams	Protein grams	Fiber grams
Lunch Totals						

Dinner	Quantity	Calories	Fat grams	Carb grams	Protein grams	Fiber grams
Dinner Totals						

Weight

Total 8 oz. glasses of water today:

Snacks	Quantity	Calories	Fat grams	Carbs grams	Protein grams	Fiber grams
Snack Totals						

Vitamins, Meds and other Supplements

		Calories	Fat grams	Carbs grams	Protein grams	Fiber grams
GRAND TOTALS > DAY#						

Physical Fitness

Type	Hours	Reps/Sets	Intensity	Calories Burned

	Bad									Excellent
My Attitude	1	2	3	4	5	6	7	8	9	10
On Track?	1	2	3	4	5	6	7	8	9	10
Belief Meter	1	2	3	4	5	6	7	8	9	10

_____
Day #

Beans are an excellent source of protein, fiber and carbohydrates.

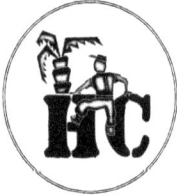

Breakfast	Quantity	Calories	Fat grams	Carb grams	Protein grams	Fiber grams
Breakfast Totals						
Lunch	Quantity	Calories	Fat grams	Carb grams	Protein grams	Fiber grams
Lunch Totals						
Dinner	Quantity	Calories	Fat grams	Carb grams	Protein grams	Fiber grams
Dinner Totals						

M = Morning
A = Afternoon
E = Evening

Weight

Total 8 oz. glasses
of water today:

Snacks	Quantity	Calories	Fat grams	Carbs grams	Protein grams	Fiber grams
Snack Totals						

Vitamins, Meds and other Supplements

		Calories	Fat grams	Carbs grams	Protein grams	Fiber grams
GRAND TOTALS > DAY#						

Physical Fitness

Type	Hours	Reps/Sets	Intensity	Calories Burned

	Bad									Excellent
My Attitude	1	2	3	4	5	6	7	8	9	10
On Track?	1	2	3	4	5	6	7	8	9	10
Belief Meter	1	2	3	4	5	6	7	8	9	10

_____ _____
Date   Day of the week

_____
Day #

One cup of cooked pasta has 200 calories. Add the sauce and an extra cup and you've got 800 - 1,200 calories.

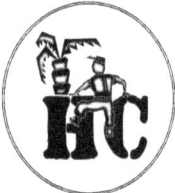

Breakfast	Quantity	Calories	Fat grams	Carb grams	Protein grams	Fiber grams
Breakfast Totals						

Lunch	Quantity	Calories	Fat grams	Carb grams	Protein grams	Fiber grams
Lunch Totals						

Dinner	Quantity	Calories	Fat grams	Carb grams	Protein grams	Fiber grams
Dinner Totals						

M = Morning A = Afternoon E = Evening	Weight		Total 8 oz. glasses of water today:			

Snacks	Quantity	Calories	Fat grams	Carbs grams	Protein grams	Fiber grams
Snack Totals						

Vitamins, Meds and other Supplements

		Calories	Fat grams	Carbs grams	Protein grams	Fiber grams
GRAND TOTALS > **DAY#**						

Physical Fitness

Type	Hours	Reps/Sets	Intensity	Calories Burned

	Bad									Excellent
My Attitude	1	2	3	4	5	6	7	8	9	10
On Track?	1	2	3	4	5	6	7	8	9	10
Belief Meter	1	2	3	4	5	6	7	8	9	10

_____ _____
Date   Day of the week

Day #

One cup of chopped broccoli has 25 calories. Compare a cup of pasta with 200 calories.

Breakfast	Quantity	Calories	Fat grams	Carb grams	Protein grams	Fiber grams
Breakfast Totals						

Lunch	Quantity	Calories	Fat grams	Carb grams	Protein grams	Fiber grams
Lunch Totals						

Dinner	Quantity	Calories	Fat grams	Carb grams	Protein grams	Fiber grams
Dinner Totals						

M = Morning
A = Afternoon
E = Evening

Weight

Total 8 oz. glasses
of water today:

Snacks	Quantity	Calories	Fat grams	Carbs grams	Protein grams	Fiber grams
Snack Totals						

Vitamins, Meds and other Supplements

		Calories	Fat grams	Carbs grams	Protein grams	Fiber grams
GRAND TOTALS > DAY#						

Physical Fitness

Type	Hours	Reps/Sets	Intensity	Calories Burned

	Bad									Excellent
My Attitude	1	2	3	4	5	6	7	8	9	10
On Track?	1	2	3	4	5	6	7	8	9	10
Belief Meter	1	2	3	4	5	6	7	8	9	10

Calorie Burn Chart I

Beverages

	Smoothie, Ban. Berry, 16 oz	Caramel Frappucino, 16 oz.	Red wine, 5 oz	Beer, 12 oz.	Orange Juice, 12 oz.	Soft drink, 12 oz.
	Jamba Juice	Starbucks	Generic	Generic	Generic	Generic
	518 cal.	**380 cal.**	**125 cal.**	**278 cal.**	**140 cal.**	**150 cal.**
Aerobics Active	65 min	48 min	16 min	35 min	18 min	19 min
Walking 3 mph	95 min	70 min	23 min	51 min	26 min	28 min
Jogging 5 mph	65 min	48 min	16 min	35 min	18 min	19 min
Biking Leisure	115 min	85 min	28 min	62 min	31 min	34 min
Dancing Energetic	80 min	59 min	20 min	43 min	22 min	23 min

Breads & Pastries

	Bagel plain	White Bread, slice	Croissant, plain	Dinner Roll	Muffin Blueberry	Scone, Blueberry
	Einstein's	Generic	Starbucks	Generic	Einstein's	Starbucks
	260 cal.	**80 cal.**	**440 cal.**	**87 cal.**	**480 cal.**	**460 cal.**
Aerobics Active	33 min	10 min	55 min	11 min	60 min	58 min
Walking 3 mph	47 min	70 min	80 min	16 min	87 min	84 min
Jogging 5 mph	33 min	10 min	55 min	11 min	60 min	58 min
Biking Leisure	58 min	18 min	98 min	20 min	107 min	102 min
Dancing Energetic	40 min	12 min	68 min	14 min	74 min	71 min

Calorie Burn Chart II

Fast Food

	Pizza Slice 3.6 oz cheese	Big Mac	French Fries large	Spagetti w/ Meat Balls 18.9 oz	Turkey Breast Wrap	5 Chicken Wings
	Generic	McDonald's	McDonald's	Pizza Hut	Subway	Hooters
	272 cal.	540 cal.	500 cal.	850 cal.	270 cal.	866 cal.
Aerobics Active	35 min	70 min	65 min	107 min	35 min	110 min
Walking 3 mph	55 min	100 min	90 min	155 min	50 min	160 min
Jogging 5 mph	35 min	70 min	65 min	107 min	35 min	110 min
Biking Leisure	60 min	120 min	115 min	190 min	60 min	200 min
Dancing Energetic	45 min	85 min	80 min	130 min	40 min	135 min

Fruit

	Apple medium	Banana medium	Raisins 4 oz	Strawberries 4 oz	Orange medium	Blueberries 4 oz
	72 cal.	105 cal.	340 cal.	36 cal.	64 cal.	45 cal.
Aerobics Active	9 min	13 min	43 min	5 min	8 min	5 min
Walking 3 mph	13 min	19 min	62 min	7 min	12 min	8 min
Jogging 5 mph	9 min	13 min	43 min	5 min	8 min	5 min
Biking Leisure	16 min	23 min	75 min	8 min	14 min	10 min
Dancing Energetic	11 min	16 min	52 min	6 min	10 min	7 min

Calorie Burn Chart III

Vegetables

	White Potato medium	Carrots Cup, grated	Peas cup	String beans cup	Spinach cup	Sweet Potato medium
	164 cal.	52 cal.	117 cal.	34 cal.	7 cal.	103 cal.
Aerobics Active	20 min	7 min	15 min	4 min	1 min	13 min
Walking 3 mph	30 min	10 min	21 min	5 min	1 min	13 min
Jogging 5 mph	20 min	7 min	15 min	4 min	1 min	13 min
Biking Leisure	36 min	12 min	26 min	8 min	2 min	23 min
Dancing Energetic	25 min	8 min	18 min	5 min	1 min	16 min

Nuts, Beans and Rice

	Almonds Dry roasted cup	Walnuts Cup, chopped	Peanuts Dry roasted cup	Black beans cup	White Rice cup	Brown Rice cup
	546 cal.	785 cal.	854 cal.	280 cal.	242 cal.	218 cal.
Aerobics Active	68 min	98 min	107 min	35 min	30 min	27 min
Walking 3 mph	99 min	143 min	155 min	51 min	44 min	40 min
Jogging 5 mph	68 min	98 min	107 min	35 min	30 min	27 min
Biking Leisure	121 min	174 min	190 min	62 min	54 min	48 min
Dancing Energetic	84 min	121 min	131 min	43 min	37 min	33 min

About the Author

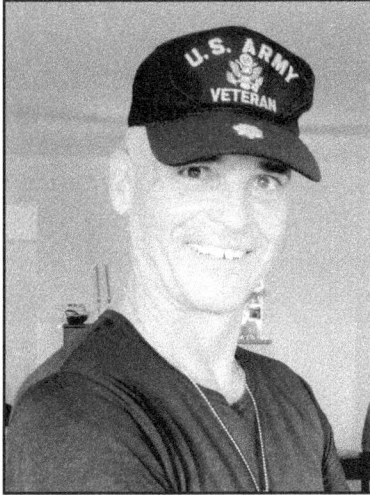

Lt. Col. Bob Weinstein, USAR-Ret.
www.TheHealthColonel.com

BIO

Born in Washington, D.C., **Lt. Col. Bob Weinstein** grew up in Virginia and spent 20 years in Berlin, Germany; he is retired from the United States Army Reserve as a Lieutenant Colonel with 30 years of service and spent about half that time as a senior military instructor with the Command & General Staff College.

He has been featured on radio and television, among others, on the History Channel and Fox Sports Net as well as in various publications such as the Washington Times, The Miami Herald and the Las Vegas Tribune.

His background is unique and diverse, including: military instructor, attorney, motivational speaker, wellness coach, certified corporate trainer, and certified personal trainer. He is fluent in German and English.

He is a popular motivational speaker at corporate events and banquets and conducts military-style workouts on Fort Lauderdale Beach utilizing strength, cardio, flexibility and agility training - both in personal training and group sessions.

He strongly believes in the importance of giving back to the community. Col. Weinstein volunteers his time for homeless and run-away kids at the Covenant House and also devotes time to training youth who are members of the US Naval Sea Cadets Corps , Team Spruance, Fort Lauderdale, Florida.

He is a member of the National Speakers Association and the American Council on Exercise.

He is the author of *Change Made Easy - Your Basic Training Orders to Excellent Physical and Mental Health.,* about personal development, fitness, exercise and health. Some of his previous clients as a guest speaker include: Sony, DHL, American Express, KPMG, AOL, IBM, AARP, SmithBarney, Green Bay Packers and Humana.

Lt. Col. Bob Weinstein, USAR-Ret.
954-636-5351
www.BeachBootCamp.net

Books and Other Products by
Lt. Col. Bob Weinstein, USAR-Ret.
www.BeachBootCamp.net

Boot Camp Fitness for All Shapes and Sizes
Paperback, $19.95, 265 pages, ISBN 978-0-9841783-1-5
EBook, $9.95, ISBN 978-0-984-17837-7 (all formats)

Weight Loss - Twenty Pounds in Ten Weeks
Paperback, $18.95, 220 pages, ISBN 978-0-9841783-0-8
EBook, $9.99, ISBN 978-0-984-17834-6 (all formats)

Quotes to Live By
Paperback, $11.95, ISBN 978-0-9841783-2-2
EBook, $5.95, ISBN 978-0-984-17833-9 (all formats)

Discover Your Inner Strength (co-author)
Paperback, $19.95
Ebook, $9.95, ISBN 978-0-984-17836-0 (all formats)

Six Keys to Permanent Weight Loss
Audio book as MP3 download (Amazon), 60 minutes
$6.93

Eight Secrets to Longevity, Health and Fitness
Audio book as MP3 download (Amazon), 50 minutes
$8.91

Health Colonel Boot Camp T-Shirts, Mugs, etc.
Go to www.cafepress.com/healthcolonel to order online

Other books by Health Colonel Publishing

The Tale of the Little Duckling by Grit Weinstein
Paperback, $14.95, picture book story for 4 to 8 year olds
ISBN 978-0-9841783-8-4
EBook, $5.99, ISBN 978-0-984-17839-1 (all formats)

"Never measure the height of a mountain until you have reached the top. Then you will see how low it was."

- Dag Hammarskjold

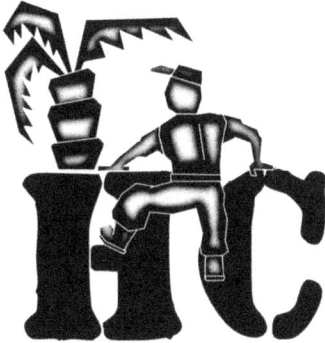

THEHEALTHCOLONEL.COM

Changing the way people think about health.

QUICK ORDER FORM

Fax orders: 866-481-2804. Send this form.

Telephone orders: Call 888-768-9892 toll-free

Email orders: thehealthcolonel@beachbootcamp.net

Postal orders: The Health Colonel, Lt. Col. Bob Weinstein, USAR-Ret., 757 SE 17th Street, #267, Fort Lauderdale, FL 33316, Telephone 954-636-5351

Please send the following books, audio CDs, DVDs:

Please send more FREE information on:

❑ Other books ❑ Speaking/seminars

❑ Fitness Boot Camp ❑ Mailing Lists

Name:

Address:

City: State: Zip:

Telephone:

Email address:

Sales tax: Please add Florida sales tax for products shipped to Florida addresses.

Shipping:
U.S.: $4.50 for first book, CD or DVD and $2.50 for each additional product.
International: $9.50 for first product; $5.50 for each additional product (estimate).

www.ingramcontent.com/pod-product-compliance
Lightning Source LLC
Chambersburg PA
CBHW030009290326
41934CB00005B/279